Disorders and Recovery

Consequences on health, as heart attack, psoriasis, acute pain, itching, dermatitis, sleep disorders, autoimmune pathology

Alex Vernocci

alexvernox editions

Table of Contents

Preface

The economic and social impact of stress and related diseases has led to consider it as the *pathology of the new century*. The biopsychosocial model (Engel, 1980), at the basis of the modern conception of health and disease, represents the epistemological matrix within which to frame stress and somatization disorders. Disorders resulting from a somatization process can affect the body in multiple forms, with effects on eating behavior, gastrointestinal (ulcers, colitis, gastritis, diarrhea), respiratory (dyspnea, hiccups, bronchial asthma), cardiovascular (hypertension, ischemia, coronary insufficiency, arrhythmia, coronary artery disease, headache migraine, tachycardia), skin (psoriasis, hyperhidrosis, eczema, rash, urticarial), musculoskeletal (cramps, arthritis, back pain, stiff neck, rheumatism psychogenic), genitourinary (menstrual pain, impotence, urination problems, incontinence), endocrine (diabetes mellitus, hyper or hypothyroidism).

Psychology and medicine have followed parallel paths almost without ever meeting for the whole last century. To attribute a so-called "psychosomatic disorder" as the cause of a strange syndrome reported by the patient represents for a doctor a sort of defeat rather than a victory. Vice versa, it will be hard for a psychologist to accept that a situation of chronic stress is able to determine an organic disease results in an almost certain loss of contact with that particular patient.

In medicine, it is emerging the awareness that the human body is not a machine, and its malfunction cannot be analyzed just by breaking the system down in its parts and by considering each of them in isolation. Neither the disease nor human behavior is predictable and they can't be modeled with a simple system based on cause-effect relationships.

This book intends to approach stress by treating it as a complex phenomenon through a multifactorial approach, which integrates the skills of different professionals engaged in caring for people affected by this problem.

By presenting evidence-based diagnostic and therapeutic techniques in a complete and updated way, this book is an exhaustive clinical guide to the diagnosis and treatment of patients with stress-related disorders.

Some main clinical pictures and related aspects of neuropsychology will be described, with a specific study dedicated to cardiovascular, gastrointestinal, and dermatological diseases, in addition to those related to sleep, to the immune system, and to eating behavior associated with weight gain.

Chapter 1 - Stress-related diseases: a general introduction

1.1 Introduction

The term "psychosomatic" first appeared in 1818, but the concept was formalized only in 1945. Over the years, the psychosomatic approach has become part of psychoanalytic theory, but today it is also claimed in the medical and scientific environments when man is considered in his concrete being, alive, sexed, acting with his own body and according to own psychic organization.

Scientists have proposed a "specific conflict model" at the origin of some psychosomatic affections, indicating that for the disturbance to occur, the concurrence of three factors is necessary: a specific conflict model, a body predisposition (factor X), and a current conflict situation. According to this view, it is the individual difference in the elaboration of emotional factors to play a pivotal role.

To date, we can still consider the coexistence of a conflictual factor and of an individual difference. Psychosomatic disorders would represent the effect of the persistence and chronicity of physiological activation due to a specific psychic conflict that prevents the discharge of emotions through action.

Psychosomatic affections dependent on blocking connected emotions of the parasympathetic activities concern various functional disorders (gastrointestinal, asthma, chronic fatigue), which constitute the outcome of a psychological and vegetative "withdrawal" of the action, and disengagement from adaptation to a hostile environment.

These studies had the merit of proposing the idea of a multifactorial approach to psychosomatic illness, where the relation among the predisposing personality, the stressful event, and the neuroendocrine mechanisms are still to be fully understood.

Bearing in mind the relevance of emotional factors, in the 70s, it has been developed the concept of "alexithymia" as a fundamental characteristic of psychosomatic patients, who are unable to "read" the emotions and express them through an abnormal and pathogenic body language.

Subsequent works have attempted to explain the complicated relationship between emotional factors and individual responses, between psyche and its expression through the soma, between organic and functional diseases.

The concept of stress eliminates the boundaries between the state of health and the state of disease, showing that there are no longer "psychosomatic illnesses" distinct from "somatic illnesses," but how any form of pathology can have, in its pathogenesis, an emotional component. To date, a significant amount of clinical-experimental data has been accumulated, and this has shown that stressful existential conditions, linked both to particular events of life and to chronic stressful events, can promote the onset of somatic diseases.

Several studies have shown how some diseases tend to develop in individuals with particular difficulties in expressing their emotional states. Subjects affected by certain diseases, which have a psychosomatic origin, such as ulcerative colitis, rheumatic arthritis, bronchial asthma etc., often have an inability to communicate their emotions.

To date, Psychosomatic Medicine is considered that part of medicine, which tends to deal more with the psychic side of illness when it is considered that the mutual influence between mind and body is essential. The relationship between emotions and somatic function is part of the concept for which the human organism is considered a physiological machine characterized not only by the biochemistry of blood but also from an emotional side that contributes to the susceptibility of the disease.

In medical practice, excluding clear cases of psychotic people and patients with organic diseases, there are many patients who do not have a serious psychopathological disorder and do not present any definite organic alteration that can explain their illness. The latter are called "purely functional." Furthermore, some patients may complain of disorders that are partly caused by emotional factors, even if some organic alterations are present, while others that suffer from ailments usually considered of pure somatic domain, but that also involve the vegetative nervous system (for example, migraine, asthma, essential hypertension).

Here are the main pathologies related to stress somatization that will be further discussed in the following paragraphs:

- Gastrointestinal complaints;

- Dermatological disorders;

- Sleep disorders;

- Pain system disorder;

- Cardiovascular disorders;

- Infertility;

- Immune system disorders.

1.2 Stress and gastrointestinal system

The digestive system is considered the part of the body most sensitive to emotions, but despite this, generally the psychic factor underlying a gastrointestinal system disorder is taken into account only in a generic way and with rather vague ideas about the nature of mental mechanisms and the role they play in determining the disease.

It is well known both from doctors and patients that emotions are a capable force to produce an alteration of the function of the digestive system, however, few are those who really care about it.

The close connection between the digestive system and emotions is explained by the dense network of fibers of the vegetative nervous system, sympathetic and parasympathetic, which act as a way of communication between the brain centers and the viscera. Also, given that the representation of how the digestive system reacts in childhood is brought back to the brain, this is deposited in memories by becoming part of the unconscious sphere.

When certain stimuli reappear, without the subject being aware of it, these memories can be projected from the unconscious to the outside, through the autonomic nervous system, reproducing the same infantile reaction pattern.

It is possible to say, for example, that the sense of security and nutrition function have a close relationship in the unconscious psyche, so when such security becomes threatened (perhaps due to stressful factors), the system that regulates nutrition can be disturbed in its normal function.

Scientists came to the conclusion that the gastrointestinal

tract, because of its three main functions, namely assumption, assimilation, and elimination of food, is particularly suitable for expressing elementary emotional tendencies, especially when the possibility of physiological expression is inhibited through the voluntary motor system.

In fact, it seems that gastric disorders are conditioned by repressed assimilation and aggressive tendencies, which are considered as chronic psychic stimuli for the gastric function. Numerous other studies have observed how psychosomatic disorders of gastrointestinal function were present in healthy subjects subjected to unusual emotional tension, becoming part of the most common manifestations of emotional tension in neurotics.

From this point of view, despite the vastness of organic disorders, we should not underestimate the ever increasing percentage of functional disorders affecting the gastrointestinal system. This perspective must lead to considering functional diagnosis not only as a diagnosis by "exclusion" but rather a diagnosis based on very precise characteristics. In other words, neurosis has its characteristic symptoms that must be sought through a careful study of personality. From this point of view, the study of the patient's personality assumes the same importance as laboratory investigations.

This applies not only in those cases in which evident signs that an anatomical lesion can be excluded but also for those that have associated clear signs of somatic illness and emotional disturbances. Just as it is not possible to overlook any potential organic injury in the so-called purely functional forms, it is even more necessary to consider the emotional side in patients who present clear signs of organic injury. In this perspective, on every type of personality, from the well-adapted to the psychotic one, psychosomatic disorders of the gastrointestinal tract can occur to these patients.

Despite the diagnostic progress, the most controversial aspect debated to date is the study of the causes and mechanism of action of peptic ulcer. In fact, despite the important contribution in the discovery in the early 80s of the *Helicobacter Pylori*, for the explanation of the development of the gastric and duodenal ulcer, the role of psychic factors should not be underestimated.

From the studies it is still unclear the relationship between stress and peptic ulcer, however from the observations made, it seems that the phenomena of chronic stress are more relevant than acute stress; so it seems that t is more relevant a large amount of small and medium difficulties of daily life, compared to a great emotional impact that rarely happens in life and that the organism is able to manage.

Currently, it has been widely accepted that gastrointestinal ailments are the result of a complex, mutual interaction of biological, psychological, and social factors that can predispose, precipitate, and perpetuate the disturbance itself. In particular, is now known the relationship with psychological disorders such as disorders of anxiety and mood.

In fact, the medicine of the twentieth century often had to face with disorders and symptoms that do not find an organic explanation, despite the innumerable instrumental investigations. In these cases, it is used the term "functional somatic disturbance."

The currently modern psychosomatic medicine is studying the complex interaction between psychological processes, physiological (physical) functions, and generation of symptoms. Through brain imaging research has in part clarified the mechanisms by which psychosocial factors could act on gastrointestinal disorders or their symptoms, even if the exact nature of this relationship remains a controversial point.

It should also be noted that somatization is a common occurrence in general medicine, and it is more common than anxiety and depression. While only a minority of somatoform patients also have anxiety and depression, most patients with depression and anxiety have a significant degree of somatization. In this case, the recognition of depression and anxiety could hinder somatic presentation.

However, somatization management cannot only involve recognition of anxiety and depression but also has to face some anxiety about the health that can be the bases for hypochondria. Ultimately, it is considered important to implement in this study a biopsychosocial integrated approach, so the 20th-century medicine should implement a holistic approach, despite technological and instrumental innovation.

1.3 Stress and sleep disturbances

Especially when insomnia is not associated with pain, with injury to the nervous system, or to some type of organic disease, it must be considered as a neurotic symptom and should be treated as a disorder from emotional conflicts.

It is known that an acute state of anxiety can disturb sleep, even if usually insomnia is not the only symptom, although it is usually the most manifest and annoying. Insomnia is difficult to diagnose as it often goes unnoticed and can happen only for a very limited period. In addition, the evaluation of insomnia is entirely subjective, given that the quantity and quality of restful sleep varies from individual to individual.

Hardly the lack of well-being during daily activities is believed to be a consequence of disturbed sleep at night. The main question is about the restorative ability of sleep rather than on the amount of sleep, as having a non-restorative sleep means that the subject is engaged in a ruminant mental activity, inability to relax, and to recover.

Therefore, insomnia mostly concerns the subjective suffering that derives from it and the degree of impairment of the subject's well-being during the day. Beyond the presence of a psychiatric disorder (mostly an anxiety disorder) or an organic disorder, most people who suffer from insomnia do not find a clinical diagnosis that explains. In sleepless individuals, the increased level of psycho-physiological activation (hyper-arousal) and the concomitant factors and mechanisms involved in the pathogenesis of hyper vigilance of the vegetative system (heart rate variability, metabolism, and skin conductance) make them particularly susceptible to stress; furthermore, all the stress systems of the central, peripheral and humoral neurons are excessively activated.

Studies show that people with insomnia tend to suffer from psychophysiological hyper-excitation, which prevents physical and mental relaxation, so they are more susceptible to stress and excessive activation of the nervous system. Moreover, in 50% of cases, they suffer from the psychological disorder (anxiety and depression), and in 10-20% of cases, insomnia must be addressed through a path of psychotherapy, also because the use of hypnotic drugs should be used just for a limited time and just for cases of acute insomnia.

Finally, it has to be considered that persistent sleep disturbances represent themselves a risk factor for cardiovascular, neuro-psychic, and gastrointestinal diseases, as well as greater mortality through interference mechanisms with the activity of the autonomous nervous system, the hypothalamus-pituitary-adrenal gland axis, and the immunological system.

1.4 Stress and dermatological diseases

If it is true that the emotions are in close relationship with the soma as they are exercising a direct influence on it, we can't avoid taking into consideration the role of the skin in this relationship. This is because it has an important symbolic meaning: the dermis represents for the individuals the fundamental point of contact between the internal world and the external one, so the skin deals with the defense of the organism from external attacks, maintaining its balance.

Psychoanalysis also explained the importance of the skin in building identity, while developmental psychology has highlighted the psychopathological consequences of an excessive stimulation of the skin or, conversely, of a poor contact.

In reality, the role of the skin as a means of expression of the inner world of the subject is also recognized in common language: in fact, it is often described with adjectives such as "bright" or "dull" which, in some way, indicate internal states of vitality or apathy. Likewise, quite common reactions like blushing or paling are the expression of the emotional states of the individual.

Despite the controversial positions that followed one another in the medical field during the twentieth century, it seems universally recognized today that some psychological components can contribute to the starting of dermatological diseases, more or less relevant. In fact, these pathologies are mediated by the immunological system of the body, as stressors act on this system through the action of the neuroendocrine network. Alongside with predisposing genetic factors, stress is considered both an antecedent of dermatological diseases and also a fundamental element in maintaining the pathological condition. More precisely, environmental factors and emotional disturbances can be considered stressors.

In addition, the severity and the recovery process for these diseases are significantly influenced by the level of social support perceived and by the coping strategies adopted from the patients. It is important to emphasize that itching and associated skin lesions are evident elements that can imply a significant reduction of the quality of life, and they appear to be frequently associated with psychiatric symptoms.

The psychosomatic pathologies affecting the skin can be divided into three main categories:

- The first one includes those conditions which, although observable at a physical level, are the strict expression of complex discomforts of psychological origin (artifact dermatitis, trichotillomania, neurotic grazes, cutaneous phobias, glossodynia and glossopyrosis, psychogenic purple syndrome);

- The second category includes chronic urticaria, generalized itching, anus-genital itching, aerated alopecia, hyperhidrosis, atopic dermatitis;

- The third group includes seborrheic dermatitis and acne, lichen planus, recurrent herpes simplex, and psoriasis.

The second and third categories include those pathologies that, although having an organic basis, are strongly influenced by psychological factors. We will examine researches relating to the most common diseases mentioned before: chronic urticaria, atopic dermatitis, and psoriasis.

1.4.1 Chronic urticaria

Urticaria is one of the most common dermatitis, and it is clinically characterized by a small lump often accompanied by itching and swelling. When urticaria becomes chronic, it is characterized by the presence of phases of decrease and increase of the symptoms that can alternate unpredictably for months or years.

Much research supports the hypothesis that psychological factors intervene in the etiology of chronic urticaria, and stressful events can be found in almost all examined patients. Since the eighties, it has been found that 90% of patients with chronic urticaria patients had been exposed to stressful events before the onset of the disease, and they suffered from psychopathological disorders (anxiety, depression), to a significantly greater extent than the other subjects participating in the study. In 2008, other scientists highlighted that psychological stress plays an important role in increasing dermatological diseases; consequently, they suggested relaxation therapies and stress management programs to reduce the impact of chronic urticaria.

1.4.2 Atopic dermatitis

Atopic dermatitis is a chronic skin disorder characterized by itching and injuries, which begins in the neonatal period or in childhood and may persist into adulthood.

The observations on the mother-child interaction highlighted the importance of this relationship in the development of pathology in the first months of life. Psychoanalysis has highlighted the presence of a mother with feelings of inadequacy with respect to her own ability to take care of the child and unable to meet her child's contact needs.

Even stress, however, seems to play an important role in the etiology of this disorder. Indeed, it appears that atopic dermatitis arises in response to stress, and that implies autonomic nervous system disorders. Patients with this disease show an excessive reactivity of the sympathetic system and itching, while the parasympathetic tone is persistently and rigidly elevated, showing a lack of adaptability in the stress response. In addition, atopic dermatitis seems to lead to a vicious circle in which the possibility of being increasingly exposed to psychological stress due to social isolation. In fact, both children and adults with atopic dermatitis show anxiety, depressive mood, and emotional excitability.

The most effective therapeutic approaches have proven to be the one associate that associate a medical treatment with psychotherapy, aimed at identifying uncomfortable situations of stress. Even behavioral relaxation techniques have proven to reduce the itching and scratching present in atopic dermatitis.

1.4.3 Psoriasis

Psoriasis is a chronic skin disease that can be associated with problems of body image and self-esteem. Therefore, this pathology has a significant emotional impact on the patient, often independently from the real severity of the condition. Such emotional stress entails an aggravation of the disease, in addition to the onset of insecurity, sexual dysfunction, anxiety, and depression, until the idea of committing suicide.

Stress, however, is not recognized only as an influencing factor for the psoriasis, but also as an element capable of playing a fundamental role in the etiology of the disease. This is especially true for type II psoriasis, which occurs after the age of 40; the type I psoriasis would instead be mainly determined by genetic factors. Research has shown how the proportion of patients with psoriasis whose disease is affected by stressful events ranging from 40 to 80%, depending on whether it is acute or chronic stress.

It was also noted in 2010 that patients with psoriasis Type II patients showed, if subjected to MMPI-2 test, characterized personality profiles with high scores on scales D (Depression), Hs (Hypochondria), Hy (Hysteria). People with this profile often have psychosomatic reactions that are the result of prolonged physiological reactions as consequences of experiences with negative emotions.

These individuals tend to use maladaptive coping strategies when they face stressful events. Consequently, the best approach for the treatment of psoriasis seems to be the one that associated with the classic medical approach also some psychotherapies that help the subject to identify situations of discomfort and to manage stress.

1.5 Other relevant clinical pictures

1.5.1 Pain system disorder

It is so called a disorder characterized by intense pain, so severe to require clinical attention, which causes significant discomfort in social functioning, work, or other areas of the patient's life. It is estimated that some psychological factor plays a role in the onset, degree of severity, increase, and maintenance of pain.

Furthermore, the symptom is not intentionally produced or simulated and cannot be explained by other types of disturbances. The subject is completely absorbed by the painful manifestations that worsen his quality of life, as pain triggers a number of negative mechanisms that relegate the individual to the role of the patient (unemployment, isolation, drug addiction).

Also, in this case, the diagnosis is usually made excluding a physical disorder that can justify the pain, and the finding of stressful psychosocial agents can help to better explain such disorder. The diagnosis is often supported by the finding of a metaphorical sense in the symptom (for example, if the patient has a back pain, this can be caused by the fact "he has been stabbed back," therefore betrayed by someone, or "he is carrying an unbearable burden"). The patient usually accepts with difficulty the presence of psychosocial stressors that act on the pain he is trying, continually seeking a physical cause for a disorder that can be non-physical.

1.5.2 Cardiac disorders

The first studies on the association between ischemic disease and "external" factors date back to the 50s, where consumption of fats, salt, and cigarette smoke were indicated as some of the most serious risks for this disease. More recently, some attention was paid to the "internal" mechanisms of response to stress, as the "context-dependent effects."

Common expressions such as "broken heart," "the heart gave out," "the heart did not withstand the stress," etc., tend to associate stress with a phenomenon of body fatigue.

By providing disadvantageous conditions and sudden physical fatigue to laboratory guinea pigs, scientists identified common sequences classifiable in the first instance as an emotional syndrome, from fear to joy, to tension, to aggressiveness. The guinea pigs presented the classic symptoms of an alarm reaction, as a profound alteration of mood, with a clear trend of adaptation of the animal's organism, to a higher threshold of response to external stimulus.

The persistence of the stressful stimulation entailed an irreversible modification in the body. At the reappearance of the alarm signal (stimulus) the guinea pig showed that it can no longer adapt and that it has exhausted its strength and died.

In fact, stressful events seem to significantly affect the cardiovascular diseases, as some epidemiological studies have found that serious loss events are associated with an increased risk of cardiovascular mortality for six months, up to six times compared to other people in the same area, age, and gender.

Other stressful events which increase the risk of having heart problems are divorce and living alone, compared to being married and living in family. In this sense, social support appears to have a positive mediation effect on cardiovascular morbidity.

It is not the stress the factor of risk, but a series of emotional conditions that accompany it. When stress is not experienced as negative, for example, in the case of a satisfactory job, it rarely leads to disorders of this type. One of the most serious effects of stress seems to be the increase in blood pressure.

Hypertension increases the risk of ischemic heart disease, and it also entails an overload of work for the heart, which increases his volume, and it atrophies. The main consequences of this overload are inadequate blood supply to the heart and the lower volume of blood circulating by contraction.

Different environmental factors can be decisive in the development of hypertension, and this increase in blood pressure has been found to be more frequent in subjects whose daily work requires permanent and high emotional tension and concentration. In addition, hypertension is more frequent in people that hold important positions and are unable to fulfill and are afraid to fail.

One of the main risk factors for cardiovascular diseases is cigarette smoke. There is a close relationship between psychic tension and smoking: when you have to pass a demanding test or expect an event of a certain importance, or you come across an unnerving discussion, the amount of consumed cigarettes increases significantly.

While experiencing stress, a general status of tension is also associated, and this is positive for the subject up to a certain threshold, as it can give him sufficient power to act effectively. Beyond that level, the tension becomes annoying and almost unsustainable. The individual is no longer able to contain it or channel it in a useful way, so he begins to leak his state by acting in various behaviors, for example, by lighting one cigarette after another.

It becomes difficult to tolerate the excess of tension both for those who suffer from it and for those who stay close to him, as proven by the large consumption of tranquilizers and sleeping pills that indicates the current state of general tension.

1.5.3 Infertility

In the last sixty years, various phenomena concerning male fertility have been detected. In fact, an alteration was found in the parameters concerning the quantity of spermatic fluid, the number of spermatozoa, and their motility, which conditions the fertility coefficient. Despite recent andrology research, many of the elements responsible for infertility remain unknown.

Among the main factors that can adversely affect the amount of sperm, it can't be excluded stress and the changed sleep-wake relationship, which act on the whole organism and therefore also on the apparatus responsible for reproduction.

Many researches have investigated the impact of stress on female fertility, and three main hypotheses have been defined:

1. Psychosocial issues have a negative impact on fertility;

2. Infertility involves the increase of stress;

3. Stress and infertility interact with each other in a reciprocal way, but such a relationship has not been completely clarified yet.

1.5.4 Immune system

Stress is one of the factors that influence the collapse of the immune condition that leads to the neoplasm. The increasing frequency of development of malignancies in Countries with high technological and industrial development makes cancer be regarded as a "stress disease," and therefore, psychosomatic.

In patients with breast cancer, it has seen a high percentage of women frustrated as mothers, in particular of women who have suffered severe trauma due to the loss or removal of a son. The tumor would have affected a part of the body believed, symbolically, as superfluous, in order to awaken a maternal function.

Emblematic is the study related to 40 patients with breast cancer that has highlighted the presence of three main characteristics, namely: a masochistic structure of character, an inhibited sexuality, and an inability to properly unload or treat hostility. Other authors have highlighted an internalized self-destructive drive in the cancer patient.

Chapter 2 - Stress and sleep disorders

2.1 Introduction

Stress is a daily aspect of the life of all individuals and is associated with negative events that can affect physical and mental health. It is often referred to a threat or danger, whether real or implied, to the body's homeostasis. In this sense, the stress response is often defined as the set of physiological and behavioral activations that are implemented by an organism to deal with it that tend to alter the homeostatic balance.

The changes that the individual must implement to respond to a stressful situation, such as adaptation to environmental stress, is sustained by systems with a high level of integration, whose adaptive response, called allostasis (the ability to maintain the stability of physiological systems by means of change), is characterized by systemic and behavioral changes aimed at developing the better homeostatic capacity of the individual, increasing his chances of survival. Allostasis is generated by the joint activity of the Central Nervous System (CNS) and the Autonomous one (ANS), the Hypothalamic-Pituitary-Adrenal (HPA) axis, the Adrenal Medullary System (AMS), and the immune-pro-inflammatory system, and uses chemical mediators such as adrenaline, glucocorticoids (cortisol) and cytokines (or interleukins, IL) that act on specific receptors located in different organs and apparatuses.

Allostasis is a process designed to maintain homeostasis, that is "maintaining stability through change," which makes the body vital and functional, allowing rapid adaptation to changing environmental conditions.

Maintaining the condition of allostasis has a cost, because when the allostatic response persists over time, as in chronic stress, it is possible to produce the so-called "allostatic load," characterized by an increased activity of the mediators on their target cells, leading to desensitization phenomena and tissue damages.

The long-term effects of the allostatic load are dramatic for the individual, such as insomnia, mental disorders (depression and anxiety), and various somatic pathologies, particularly affecting the cardiovascular and respiratory systems.

2.2 Molecular, hormonal and inflammatory aspects of stress

The brain plays a key role in the evaluation of potentially stressors events, but it is also the preferential target of the action of the mediators of stress, especially glucocorticoids and cytokines. The brain's response to stress, regardless of whether it is acute or chronic, must be included in the chapter of adaptive plasticity.

Recent studies on hippocampal creation have provided specific evidences of how neuronal plasticity is regulated by hormone levels and immune system activity/inflammation, both in adult life and during development. The discovery that glucocorticoid receptors are abundantly expressed in hippocampal formation has led many researchers to focus their attention right on the hippocampus as a target region of stress.

It has been widely described in literature that chronic stress is associated with high levels of glucocorticoid and with specific interleukin levels, which alter themselves both the structure and the hippocampal function.

From a morphological point of view, the consequences of hormonal alteration and inflammatory condition induce the reduction of the hippocampal volume, which implies some dendritic atropism and reduction of neurogenesis, i.e., the capacity to form new neurons. It has been indeed shown that treatment with inhibitors of glucocorticoid prevents stress-related dendritic atrophy, indicating how endogenous glucocorticoids are the main culprits of morphological consequences of stress in the brain.

Functionally, chronic stress is generally associated with the reduction of excitability of the hippocampus and the long-term potentiation mechanisms (LTP, Long Term Potentiation), whose main consequence is represented by alterations of the hippocampal memory function.

It has recently been hypothesized that the pathophysiological mechanism responsible for some mental disorders associated with stress, such as depression and Post-Traumatic Stress Disorder (PTSD), is due to a loss of neurons or to the alteration of hippocampal neurogenesis.

This hypothesis finds its rationale in the negative effects on both neurogenesis and dendritic tropism induced by the increase of plasma in the cortisol levels, and some inflammatory interleukins that are typically found to be increased in depression and PTSD.

The advent of "endo-phenotype" has also introduced a new aspect of the response to stress: the individual multifactorial genetic differences can play a crucial role in making subjects more or less vulnerable to negative effects to chemical stress mediators. Recently it was posed great attention to some polymorphisms associated with the serotonergic system functioning and to the expression of the cortisol receptors, and to some growth factors as BDNF.

2.3 Basic aspects of the interaction between sleep and stress

Sleep deprivation or sleep restriction is an example of allostatic load, as both conditions lead to alterations that are typical of stress and are conditions that can trigger stress, such as depression. It has been highlighted as the destruction of sleep, or its chronic restriction may selectively interfere with the activity of the hippocampus, going to inhibit neurogenesis and contribute, at least partially, to the etiology of depression.

It is also sufficient to remember how the deprivation of a single night of sleep has an effect, albeit weak, on the basal rate of proliferation and cellular survival at the hippocampal level. Despite the extensive literature on this, the neurobiological mechanisms by which sleep deprivation influences hippocampal neurogenesis are to date partially unknown.

It has been proposed that the inhibitory effect of deprivation of sleep on neurogenesis may be supported by an indirect effect linked to an increase of the stress levels, in particular glucocorticoids. In this regard, it has been observed that:

- Prolonged sleep fragmentation is associated with changes in the regulation of the HPA axis similar to those observed in depression;

- Low level of plasmatic glucocorticoid levels may prevent suppression of hippocampal neurogenesis induced by sleep deprivation. On the other hand, some studies conducted with adrenaline rats have recently shown that prolonged sleep loss can inhibit hippocampal neurogenesis independently from the increase of glucocorticoids.

Many other factors can be modulated and influenced by sleep deprivation, and some of these could represent the missing ring between sleep deprivation and reduced neurogenesis. It has been proven, for example, how the reduction of neurogenesis following sleep deprivation could be related to an increase in plasma or central levels of inflammatory interleukins.

Both interleukin 6 (IL-6) and tumor necrosis factor-alpha (TNF) increase after sleep restrictions; elevated plasma levels of IL-6 are commonly found in patients suffering from primary insomnia and depression. Studies in vitro have identified that both IL-6 and TNF decrease neurogenesis, suggesting how these cytokines can at least partially mediate some of the negative effects of neuro-inflammation on in vivo hippocampal neurogenesis.

2.4 Psychophysiological and pathophysiological aspects of the interaction between sleep and stress

Although the association between sleep and stress is well known, a more systematic and scientific approach emerged only from the 80s, when it has been demonstrated that the Slow Wave Sleep (SWS, stages 3 and 4 of sleep NREM) represents one of the specific stress targets.

Initially, the relationships between the HPA axis (hypothalamic CRH, pituitary ACTH, and adrenal cortisol) and sleep emerged from studies modulating the activity of the axis in the absence of stressful conditions. In the animal model, it has been observed that the administration of CRH induces an increase in the waking state, thanks to an excitatory effect on different subcortical structures such as the locus coeruleus (region of the activating reticular system, hyperactive during wakefulness), the amygdala, the hippocampus, and some hypothalamic nuclei.

In experimental human models, the administration of CRH or synthetic glucocorticoids induces an increase in arousal levels, with neuro-vegetative hyperactivity and reduction of deep sleep. The increase in arousal levels is associated with an increase in the expression of high electroencephalographic frequencies, and therefore to fragmentation and reduction of sleep.

According to these considerations, some works show a significant correlation between cortisol levels, stress, and number of nocturnal arousal, as well as of an inverse correlation between Slow Wave Activity (SWA, spectral band power in band-delta) and cortisol levels during NREM sleep.

Furthermore, the effects of CRH seem to be age-dependent: it has been demonstrated that sleep in young individuals is relatively resistant to the effect of CRH, while middle-aged individuals respond to CRH administration with a more marked reduction in the SWA and an increase in the sleep alarm. Therefore, it is possible to speculate that increasing age makes subjects more vulnerable to manifest a greater instability of deep night sleep, and this could explain the highest incidence of insomnia in this population group.

The effects of cortisol on sleep appear more complex than they can be superimposed by some direct effects mediated by two types of receptors (GR for glucocorticoids, MR for mineralocorticoids) and indirect effects related to inhibitory feedback of the secretion of the CRH, as well as the time in which cortisol is administered (the cortisol is a hormone with circadian properties).

On the other hand, the data on the effects of stress on REM sleep are rather contradictory. While some studies conducted on healthy subjects have shown how acute stress exposure is associated with more frequent REM sleep disturbances compared to NREM, increasing its duration and reducing its latency, others have not detected any modification. One of the possible explanations of this inconsistency could be represented by the individual psychophysiological reactivity, therefore by the so-called coping strategies which the subject responds to the stressful event, activating the various physiological systems such as the HPA axis and the SAM (Sympathetic Adrenal Medullary) system.

Unlike what happens in acute stress, exposure to chronic stress always determines changes in REM sleep, such as an increase in the first REM period, in the density of eye movements, and in the total duration.

The changes that REM sleep is suffering seem to be of fundamental importance in connecting sleep with stress, and also with psychopathological elements of the affective sphere. In this regard, the short REM latency and the higher REM density were related to central hypertonicity cholinergic, which is believed to be an integral part of the pathophysiology of depression.

Some recent experimental evidence indicates that the pontine cholinergic structures that generate REM sleep are activated during sleep by neuronal groups belonging to the amygdala system. This structure, which plays a key role in the modulation of emotional responses, such as fear or stress, is overactive in wakefulness and in the sleep of depressed patients. If on one hand the dysfunction of the amygdala system is believed to be responsible for changes in the affective sphere, on the other hand, it could help determine REM sleep disturbances typical of the stress response (allostatic state) or depressive pathology (allostatic load).

2.5 New psychophysiological aspects of slow wave sleep

Recently it has been shown how the homeostatic effects of sleep are related to slow oscillations of the membrane potential in the cortical neurons (<1Hz), which are mainly born in prefrontal regions and characterize slow wave sleep (SWS). Intracellular recording studies of the Mircea Steriade group carried out in animals that are sleeping naturally have shown that during waking, the membrane potential of cortical neurons remains stable at around −65mV. During SWS the potential becomes biphasic with harmonic oscillations between −85mV and −65mV.

This behavior has been defined by Mircea Steriade slow oscillation and represents the basic cellular phenomenon of slow-wave sleep. Slow oscillation is characterized by periods called *up-state* (duration about 500 ms), in which the neuronal and synaptic discharge activity can be superimposed both in terms of frequency and space-time coherence to the one present in REM sleep and in wakefulness, and by periods called *down-state* (duration about 500 ms) in which the deep hyperpolarization is associated to an electric cortical silence and therefore the absence of any network activity.

It is important to underline how this oscillation has a cortical origin, as it has been shown that it persists even after the removal of the thalamus, because it involves all neurons of the cortex of any layer, both inhibitors, and exciters. The slow oscillation generated at the cortical level is transmitted to subcortical structures such as the thalamus, basal prosencephalon, hippocampus, brain stem, and neostriate.

This cellular behavior has also been identified on the human EEG, and it represents the fundamental phenomenon that underlies neural activity in the SWS; in humans, slow oscillation has been called sleep slow oscillation (SSO).

Recently scientists have described the following basic SSO properties:

- It brushes the human cortex with a frequency of one per second, acting as a traveling wave;

- It has a specific source of origin, most frequently located in the anterior cortical regions (prefrontal cortex), typically spreading to the rear regions;

- It has a high reproducibility between nights and

between subjects.

In addition to these spatial and dynamic properties, a close relationship has been demonstrated between SSO and the synaptic plasticity that underlies both the implicit learning and the declarative memory. These spatial, dynamic, and functional characteristics make SSO a key phenomenon to quantify sleep quality and to characterize some of its functions.

Finally, SSO seems to play a central role in the hypothesis that sees sleep as a modulator of synaptic homeostasis. According to this hypothesis, the function of the SWS would be attributable to a phenomenon of synaptic down-scaling that is the reduction of the cortical synaptic "weight," which would tend to favor the consolidation of the memory through a fine modulation of the signal/noise ratio in the cortical circuitry.

Recently, thanks to the experimental model represented by the simulation of human flight to Mars (MARS 500 project), the modulation of the stress on sleep, and in particular on SSO, in environmental conditions characterized by social and spatial confinement, high workload, shifts, and emergencies.

This model is particularly interesting as it identifies one close prenosological relationship between cortisol, sleep patterns, and certain characteristics of the structure and topology of the SSO.

It has been observed as high levels of cortisol and stress are associated with a significant reduction in recognition of the SSO, in particular in the front-central-parietal regions. In line with this data, it can be assumed that chronic exposure to stressors events associated with sleep changes (especially those related to SSO) may lead to a condition characterized by alterations in neuronal plasticity. The significant alteration of synaptic down-scaling could lead to an abnormal evolution of cortical synaptic levels during sleep and, therefore, to changes in neural mechanisms that underlie some cognitive functions, such as memory and learning.

2.6 Clinical aspects of the interaction between sleep and stress

The relationship between sleep and stress has assumed a central importance for the medicine of sleep when in the late 90s scientists reformulated insomnia "neurocognitive" theory. From a behavioral perspective, some models see acute insomnia associated with predisposing and precipitating factors (such as psychosocial stressors), and chronic perpetuating factors (such as the increase of time spent in bed).

In the context of the behavioral perspective, experiences during the day (psychosocial stress, inadequate ability to solve problems, worries, and ruminations) profoundly affect sleep, partly undermining its continuity and even more own capability to rest (acute insomnia). Over time, insomnia sufferers start to complain about the quality of their sleep, to have selective attention to everything related to sleep as well as to the more or less intense sleepiness and a series of dysfunctional disorders, both somatic and psychic.

It is a single cycle in which wakefulness and sleep are interdependent elements that lead to transient insomnia. In other words, altered sleep is more or less directly at the basis of the quality of waking, as well as a stressful vigil (mental, social and physical) is the basis of poor quality sleep.

The persistence of insomnia is associated with behavioral adaptations, such as for example, staying awake in bed, which negatively affects the evolution of the alteration of sleep up to imply a situation of chronic insomnia, which aggravates the already existing levels of daytime stress and further increase this vicious circle. It has been speculated that the basis of the evolution of insomnia there is an abnormal cortical arousal during sleep, which is expressed on the experiential side in the form of increased cognitive and instrumental activity for an increase in fast EEG activities (beta and gamma).

In the context of "neurocognitive" theory, hyper-arousal represents the result of a classic conditioning, and it promotes abnormal levels of sensory processing, of information processing, and the formation of long-term memories, thus making the sleepless subject most vulnerable to environmental stress (difficulty in falling asleep and frequent awakenings), to the distinction between sleep and wakefulness (altered sleep perception), to the consolidation of negative memories.

Therefore, it is not surprising that this model predicts that chronic insomnia increases vulnerability to affective psychopathology, in particular towards depression and anxiety disorders. What was said on the neurophysiological and biochemical level in the previous paragraphs, it also seems to be confirmed on a clinical level: stress seems to be a common factor at the bases of both insomnia and depression.

Based on the various evidences present in the literature and on the considered hypothesis of "diathesis stress" (i.e., stress produces damage where there is a specific vulnerability in the organism), insomnia as an element or expression of allostatic load can be considered an independent risk factor of depression only when it encounters a multifactorial genetic substrate with increased susceptibility to stress.

As mentioned, the clinical evidences are many, and they

indicate that for 57% of chronic insomnia, within a two-year period, there is the onset of a mood or anxiety disorder, whose incidence is more than double that of the general population (24%).

2.7 Conclusions

With this brief review, we set out the relationship between stress and sleep and their implications for the psychobiological research and clinical practice of the psychologist and psychiatrist. The main points of the relationship between sleep and stress can be summarized as follows:

1. The physiological response to stress, or allostasis, is characterized by an integrated multisystem activation that involves various systems, from the central nervous one to the autonomic, from the hypothalamic-pituitary-adrenal axis to the immune/inflammatory axis;

2. The persistence of the allostatic response, as occurs in conditions of chronic stress, induces the so-called "allostatic load," characterized by increased activity of mediators on their target cells, leading to desensitization phenomena and tissue damage, such as alterations of dendritic tropisms and hippocampal neurogenesis;

3. Chronic stress represents one of the pathophysiological elements for the development of insomnia and mental disorders, such as depression and anxiety disorders;

4. Chronic insomnia as an expression of allostatic load represents a factor of risk that is independent of the development of both mood and anxiety disorder in the presence of a specific multifactorial genetic vulnerability.

In general, subjects in allostasis conditions can be placed on the ascendant phase of a hypothetical curve, in which the peculiar hormonal/inflammatory structure of the stress tends to sustain some cognitive performances thanks to the positive effects of eustress level. This is similar to the Yerkes-Dodson curve, which describes the relationship between anxiety levels and cognitive performance.

From a purely heuristic point of view, it can be assumed that the persistence of the stress condition, and in particular of sleep disturbances, may lead to the passage in the descending phase of that curve, characterized by those emotional, cognitive, and behavioral alterations that are typical of the allostatic load.

In other words, the same mechanisms activation of the HPA axis, the sympathetic nervous system, and the immune system, which contribute to the allostatic response, can be amplified by the alteration of sleep (insomnia), which could ultimately represent one of the "catastrophic" factors to induce the transition from an allostatic state to an allostatic load.

The development of new molecular, genetic, and function investigation methodologies in vivo in humans, such as magnetic resonance imaging (MRI) and high density EEG (HiDe-EEG), offered new possibilities for studying neural correlates, both structural and functional, stress and related diseases.

For example, identifying the close relationships between hippocampal neurogenesis, genetic polymorphisms of vulnerability to stress, impaired sleep, and depression are a paradigmatic example of a translational approach from molecule to man.

Along these lines, the study of the relationships between stress and sleep slow oscillation (SSO) stands as a pioneering research, whose psychophysiological approach can find fruitful application in identifying the negative effects of stress on sleep and its functions. For example, the SSO study could find its own location in the preclinical field for the characterization and identification of multiple borderline conditions that, although without defined clinical manifestations, are conditioning the subjective vulnerability towards the development of pathologies related to stress.

This could contribute to the identification of predictive risk indexes and, therefore, of ad hoc countermeasures (such as transcranial electrical stimulation) in order to confine stress-related manifestations exclusively in the prenosological field.

On the clinical level, the observation that arises is the need to pay much more attention to stress and to disturbed sleep than paid in the last decades. In clinical psychology, the psychologist cannot ignore the sleep problems, and in particular, insomnia, as a warning symptom, an indicator of the severity of the allostatic load. On the other hand, disturbed sleep itself acts negatively as a stressor, influencing allostasis and thus causing a vicious circle in which the two alterations self-feed each other.

By adopting this conception, we will no longer consider a simple causal relationship between stress and disturbed sleep, but at a progression of the allostatic load, which can undermine the psychic balance up to contribute to the onset of a mental disorder related to the emotional sphere, such as depression and anxiety disorders.

Chapter 3 - Stress and dermatological diseases

3.1 Introduction

Skin diseases are frequent, and for psoriasis alone, for example, it has been estimated a prevalence of 2-3% in the general population of various European countries. They are pathologies that can present with various symptoms and signs such as pain, itching, burning, blistering, pigmentation, or discoloring of the skin, thickening of the skin, loss of hair or eyebrows. Lesions on the skin can be visible and damage the person's appearance or behave, till to real physical disfigurements.

It is therefore understood how such pathologies can lead to a heavy load of suffering and disability and seriously influence the lives of affected people. Some patients report experiences of stigma, and many complain of an impairment of daily activities and a deterioration in the quality of life. The reduction of psychosocial well-being does not only concern patients treated by a specialist in dermatological centers, but even those assisted in general medicine.

Skin pathologies represent one of the main areas of clinical activity and research in psychosomatic medicine. There are various important links between skin and mind, and this is explaining the growing interest of psychosomatics for these diseases. The skin and central nervous system are related from the embryological point of view for their common origin from the ectoderm, they share many hormones, neurotransmitters, and receptors.

The skin also plays an essential role throughout the life cycle as a sensory organ in socialization processes, it is responsive to various emotional stimuli, and its appearance can influence the body image and self-esteem. The touch of the skin between people can have an incredible emotional power, as can transmit a sense of welcome, availability, warmth, closeness, intimacy, and affection.

3.2 Psychiatric morbidity in dermatological patients

A large number of epidemiological studies have documented the frequent presence of psychiatric disorders in patients with skin diseases. For example, in a study out of 2500 patients, the prevalence of psychiatric morbidity, determined by means of the 12-item version of the General Health Questionnaire (GHQ-12), was 25%.

In another study on 600 hospitalized patients, the prevalence of psychiatric morbidity, determined through the Structured Clinical Interview for DSM-IV Disorders Axis I, was estimated at 38%. The most frequently observed disturbances were related to mood (20%) and anxiety (16%), in which the most common diagnoses are the depressive disorder (7%), the generalized anxiety disorder (6%), the dysthymic disorder (5%) and the panic disorder (4%). Even adaptation disorders and somatoform disorders have been found in many patients, with a prevalence of 7% for both diagnostic categories.

Various psychological conditions have also been observed with great of psychosomatic interest, defined according to the Diagnostic Criteria for Psychosomatic Research (DCPR), such as demoralization (14%), irritable mood (14%), type A behavior (12%), anxiety about health (11%) and alexithymia (6%). Furthermore, a non-negligible prevalence, around 2%, was observed for each of the DCPR conditions characterizing an abnormal behavior towards disease, such as nosophobia, persistent somatization, tanatophobia, conversion symptoms, and denial of the disease.

Overall, at least one condition was diagnosed in 48% of patients according to DCPR. It should be noted that almost half of these patients do not have received a DSM-IV diagnosis, and therefore they would not have been identified as patients worthy of psychiatric attention if the DCPR criteria had not been used.

The finding in these studies of a high prevalence of psychiatric morbidity is in line with the results of numerous other studies conducted in various countries, both on groups of patients with heterogeneous dermatological diagnoses and on groups of patients with specific skin pathologies such as psoriasis, acne, atopic dermatitis, alopecia aerated, urticaria, vitiligo, idiopathic pruritus, systemic sclerosis.

Various studies have shown that the localization of skin lesions on the face or hands, and in general, their visibility is associated with an increased risk of psychiatric morbidity, especially in the female sex.

An important topic concerns the not rare presence of suicidal ideation in patients with dermatological diseases:

- In a pioneering article on the subject, two dermatologists described 16 cases of patients they had visited in the past 20 years who had committed suicide, 8 of whom had acne. In a later study on 330 British dermatologists, participants reported knowing average of 178 patients who had attempted suicide and 27 who had committed suicide. This problem was then the subject of systematic epidemiological studies.

- In a study, depressive symptoms and suicidal ideation were assessed using the Carroll Rating Scale for Depression on 460 patients with various skin diseases. The prevalence of suicidal ideation determined by the "I thought to try to kill myself" item was 7.2% in hospitalized psoriatic patients, 5.6% in patients with mild or moderate facial acne, 2.5% in outpatient psoriatic patients, and 2.1% in patients with atopic dermatitis.

- In another study, on 340 outpatient dermatological patients, 170 hospitalized dermatologists patients, and 296 paired healthy subjects, a significantly higher percentage of patients with psoriasis (21.2% of 113) and atopic dermatitis (18.9% of 95) reported suicidal thoughts compared to healthy subjects (6.8%).

- In a study of 477 patients (300 outpatient and 177 hospitalized), when asked in the Patient Health Questionnaire (PHQ), "Over the past 2 weeks, with what frequency was annoyed by thinking that it would be better to be dead or think of harming yourself in any way?" about 6% of patients responded "For several days," and 3% "more than half the days" or "almost every day," for an overall prevalence of suicidal ideation of 8.6%. Even considering only outpatient patients, the prevalence of suicidal ideation was 4.8%. The validity of the evaluation of the suicidal ideation has been supported by the absence of the same in 58 patients with mild dermatological diseases, with presumed low emotional impact (moles, mycoses, keratosis, and warts), opposite of a high frequency in diseases with the greater impact such as acne (7.1%), skin tumors (8.3%), various dermatitis (8.8%), psoriasis (10%) and urticaria (18.8%).

- In the multivariate analysis, the only factors independently associated with the idea of suicide were the emotional suffering and the impairment of quality of life, measured with GHQ-12 and Skindex-29, respectively. The items most strongly associated with suicidal ideation were those related to feelings of sadness, frustration, humiliation, and difficulty in intimate relationships.

- In another study conducted in Pakistan, a 7.1% prevalence of suicidal ideation was observed in acne patients.

- Recently, some studies were carried out on samples of young acne patients recruited from the community rather than in clinical settings. In a New Zealand study on 9570 students aged between 12 and 18, there was an association between the presence of acne and suicide attempts, which has also remained significant by controlling for the severity of depressive and anxious symptoms.

- These results have been confirmed by a recent

Norwegian study of 3780 young people aged 18-19, in which almost a quarter of people with severe acne reported suicidal ideation.

- In a study conducted in Japan on 6752 patients with atopic dermatitis, the prevalence during the life of the suicidal ideation was 19.6% in more severe patients, and it was 6% in patients with moderate disease, compared to 8.1% found in 3582 healthy people.

- In another recent German study, the prevalence of suicidal ideation was significantly higher in 62 adult patients with atopic dermatitis compared to a paired group of healthy people.

- In patients with skin diseases, the presence of psychiatric morbidity has various and important correlated. First, it is associated with greater quality impairment of life. In a study of 2,142 outpatient dermatological patients, the presence of psychiatric morbidity, determined with GHQ-12, was found to be associated with a greater negative influence of skin symptoms on the quality of life in all dermatological diseases that cause perceptible symptoms such as pain, itching or burning.

- In another study, the presence of a psychiatric diagnosis DSM-IV or a DCPR condition was found to be associated with poorer quality of life in the domains of social functioning and emotions. In addition, the presence of a DCPR condition, but not of a DSM-IV diagnosis, was found to be associated with a greater impairment of quality of life by symptoms of skin disease.

- These results are consistent with those of other studies that suggested a link between the emotional state and the severity of itching and other sensory skin symptoms.

- In a longitudinal study of 389 outpatient dermatological patients, the strongest predictor of poor adherence to the prescriptions of the dermatologist was the presence of a depressive or anxiety disorder. In this study, the risk of poor adherence to treatment was about three times greater in patients with psychiatric morbidity compared to those free of psychiatric disorders.

3.3 The direction of the causal flow

Given the frequent simultaneous presence of dermatological and psychiatric morbidity, the question of what are the mutual causal relationships needs to be examined. Some cases may be attributed to the side effects of certain medications. If on one hand the side effects on the skin due to psychotropic drugs such as lithium or some antipsychotics are known, on the other, also side effects on the mood due to drugs widely used in dermatology such as corticosteroids are also well known.

In addition, in some cases, both psychiatric and skin symptoms are secondary to systemic diseases, such as lupus erythematosus or porphyria. It can also happen that the dermatologist finds himself visiting patients with a primary psychiatric disorder that has led to skin lesions, such as trichotillomania, body dysmorphic disorder, a delusional disorder with delirium of parasitosis, and some cases of obsessive compulsive disorder with skin lesions caused by repeated washing.

However, these explanations can cover only to a limited extent for the frequent simultaneous presence of dermatological and psychiatric morbidity. A hypothesis with greater explanatory potential is that the causal flow proceeds from the skin to the mind, so means that the psychiatric morbidity manifests itself as a complication of a dermatological disease, for example, in reaction to an aesthetic damage, to stigma experiences, or unwanted lifestyle changes due to skin pathology, as per the following steps:

1. Starting of a skin pathology;

2. Alteration of the body image (more severe if lesions are visible and in the genital area). Impairment of social functioning (more serious if intimate emotional relationships are affected). Unwanted lifestyle changes and reduced quality of life. Stigmatization experiences;

3. Unpleasant self-conscious emotions (embarrassment, shame). Sadness. Concern, tension;

4. Failure to improve skin pathology and persistence of the situation;

5. Consolidation of emotional suffering in a diagnosable mental disorder.

To support this hypothesis, there are numerous cross-cutting studies that highlighted the relevance of the experiences of stigma and stress secondary in the presence of dermatological pathology. A recent study of psoriasis patients suggested that a compromised quality of life caused by dermatological disease induces the raising of depressive symptoms.

These studies, although suggestive, cannot document cause-effect relationships for the limitations inherent in the transversal design. However, the hypothesis was also supported by studies with a longitudinal design. In a study on patients hospitalized for psoriasis, the patients who tested positive for psychiatric screening by GHQ-12, it has been observed an association between the occurrences of a clinical improvement relevant to skin disease and the reduction of the GHQ-12 score, that was going down below the threshold for positivity.

Clearly, together with the hypothesis of a causal flow from the skin to the mind, also the opposite hypothesis could be also be considered, so the causal influence of psychological factors, in particular the emotional stress, on the course of various skin diseases.

There are numerous studies that have been conducted to test this hypothesis, although there are relatively few that have been conducted with a sufficiently solid methodology.

Longitudinal studies have investigated the possible role of perceived stress. Two studies conducted on small samples suggested a correlation between the perceived daily stress level and the clinical course of psoriasis, and atopic dermatitis, while a longitudinal study of a group of university students under examination showed a correlation between the perceived stress level and the clinical course of acne.

Stressful life events have been subject to as much attention as possible as a potential etiological factor for some skin diseases. Various anecdotal descriptions of clinical cases and numerous observational studies not controlled in case series have suggested a relationship between the occurrence of stressful events and the appearance or increase of various skin pathologies. However, most of these studies are burdened by serious methodological limitations such as the absence of a control group and by the use of non-standardized measures of stressful events.

There are some studies with better methodological quality, with case-control design, that have documented an association between the occurrence of stressful events and the appearance or the intensification of pathologies such as psoriasis, alopecia aerated, vitiligo, and lichen planus.

However, some results were negative, and various studies have used it for the evaluation of stressful events using self-filled questionnaires, which have less reliability than evaluation tools based on an interview. Also, the studies they have controlled the influence of possible confounding factors are rare, such as discontinuation of dermatological treatment, alcohol and cigarette consumption, sun exposure, or seasonal effects.

A series of case-control studies have suggested that to better understand the controversial relationship between events, and potentially stressful situations and skin health should take into account the characteristics of people. In these studies, the cases consisted of recently outpatient patients (less than 3 months), with beginning or increasing of vitiligo (n = 31), or with recent beginning of alopecia aerate (n = 21), and from patients hospitalized with recent beginning or intensification of diffuse psoriasis plaque (n = 33).

The controls were established respectively by 116 outpatients and by 73 hospitalized patients with dermatological pathologies, believing to have a low psychosomatic component such as, for example, moles or warts. In these studies, not only the recent stressors events were investigated (last 12 months, excluding cases of subsequent events at the onset or intensification of the skin pathology) identified by means of the Paykel semi-structured interview, but also the level of social support received and some individual characteristics related to emotional regulation, such as alexithymia and attachment style.

In these analyzes, it has also been checked for other possible risk factors such as alcohol and cigarette consumption. The results of these studies were similar in the different skin pathologies studied, suggesting a minor role for stressful events, against a more important role of the social support and individual differences in emotional regulation.

A higher level of alexithymia was found to increase the risk of increasing the disease in patients with psoriasis plaque and with vitiligo, and tend to increase the risk of starting of the alopecia aerate. It was also observed that a higher level in avoidance of attachment relationships tends to increase the risk of alopecia aerate, also associated with the recent increase of plaque and curtain psoriasis to be associated with a recent aggravation of vitiligo.

It was also found that a higher level of anxiety in attachment relationships tends to increase the risk of aggravation of vitiligo. An association was also observed between receiving less perceived social support and recent intensification in patients with psoriasis plaque and vitiligo and a tendency to associate with the rise of pathology in patients with alopecia aerate.

However, no association was found between the raising or increasing of alopecia aerate, psoriasis plaque, and vitiligo, and the total number of recent stressing events or the number of serious, undesirable, or uncontrollable events. The only association found was between the exposure to three or more non-controllable events and the aggravation of vitiligo. These results have been supported by subsequent studies:

- A case-control study found an association between the increase of psoriasis and major avoidance and anxiety in attachment relationships, less social support, and the occurrence of a subset of the stressful events investigated by the Paykel interview.

- A study of 45 patients with alopecia areata compared
  with 56 healthy subjects, matched by gender and
  age, has supported the hypothesis of a role of
  alexithymia, while it has not been found any
  association with stressful events.

- Another study also observed higher levels of
  alexithymia in patients with alopecia aerate
  compared with patients with other skin diseases.

- The results of a French study suggested a link
  between a lower ability to integrate and differentiate
  emotions and reactivity to stress in patients with
  psoriasis.

- The importance of social support was confirmed by a
  study with patients with psoriasis and atopic
  dermatitis, in which psychological stress was
  associated more strictly with less social support,
  rather than with clinical severity and the physical
  symptoms of itching.

The results of these studies allow us to better articulate the
pathogenic hypothesis, which involves stress in skin
diseases. They are consistent with the theories that a
stressful condition does not simply result from a stimulus
coming from the environment, but derives from the

interaction between the environment and the person itself.

A possible causal flow from mind to skin can be summarized in the following steps:

1. Potentially stressful event or situation;

2. Rated as relevant in terms of possible harm, loss or threat or challenge, based on the organization of personal significance, individual biography, and life cycle stage;

3. Maladaptive personality traits. Reduced capacity for emotional regulation. Poor quantity and quality of social relationships that can provide support;

4. Stress;

5. Neuro-endocrine-cutaneous network, autonomic nervous system;

6. Skin tissue damage.

In fact, stressful events and situations do not act on an inert object. The emotions, thoughts, and behaviors of the person who experiences the event contribute substantially to start and keep the stressful conditions. The first step of the causal path that can lead from a life event to a skin pathology probably concerns the meaning of that event for the specific person, based on personal history, life phase, and individual personal meaning.

The importance of personal meaning in psychobiology and in psychosomatics is supported by the great inter-individual variability of the psycho-neuroendocrine response to the same potentially stressful situation. If the person perceives an event as relevant in terms of possible damage, loss, threat, or challenge, and trigger a stressful reaction in the body, other factors come into play. Among these are the quantity and quality of social relationships that can provide support and capacity, less in people with insecure attachment, to make effective use of available social support.

There are also various aspects of the emotional regulation that go from the ability to discriminate emotions and internal states, which by definition is reduced in people with high alexithymia, to the ability to effectively regulate affections and to integrate emotional and cognitive information, which is less in people with insecure attachment.

Therefore, in the presence of psychosocial factors of individual vulnerability, some specific events, and life situations can cause a particularly acute state or prolonged stress that can cause damages in the skin tissue, especially when predisposing biological factors are also present local level.

A plausible mediator in the relationship between stress and diseases of the skin is the complex neuro-endocrine-immune network. In vulnerable individuals, the release of neuro-immune substances triggered by the stress can adversely affect the skin homeostasis through the activation of inflammatory processes in the deeper layers.

Furthermore, psychological stress damages the scarring response of the skin and alters the permeability barrier at the epidermis level, which may facilitate the development or persistence of skin, inflammatory conditions.

Overall, data from the relatively few studies conducted on causals relationship between mind and skin support the hypothesis that the flow of causality may proceed both from skin to mind and from mind to skin. The causal link between dermatological and psychiatric morbidity, therefore, appears to be, in all probability, bidirectional, although there is still much to understand about it.

3.4 Management of the dermatological patient in a psychosomatic perspective

The high prevalence of mental disorders and conditions of psychosomatic interest among patients with skin diseases requires that appropriate clinical attention is dedicated to the psychosocial aspects in these patients, also in considering the high risk of self-injurious behavior, greater emotional distress, worse quality of life, and reduced adherence to dermatological treatment.

Most patients with psychiatric comorbidity come to the observation of the dermatologist before consulting a mental health specialist: dermatologists therefore have a key role in identifying and treating, or start treatment, the psychiatric morbidity of their patients.

Dermatologists are generally very competent in recognizing psychopathology in patients with a mental disorder that presents a dermatological problem. Classic examples are trichotillomania, the rare Ekbom syndrome or delirium of parasitoids, and self-inflicted skin lesions.

It seems less satisfactory, instead, the recognition of mental disorders in patients with real skin diseases. In a study of 292 outpatient dermatological patients in which the psychic state had been assessed both with standardized questionnaires and independently by the dermatologist, two thirds of cases of probable depressive disorder or anxiety have not been recognized by dermatologists. This result is in line with two other English studies that also found a frequent failure in recognizing mental disorders in daily dermatological practice.

These studies suggest that in many clinical settings, the high workload and the limited time available for each visit make it difficult for dermatologists to pay sufficient attention to the mental health needs of their patients.

To improve the situation, various initiatives can be put in place, for example, specific training programs for the recognition and management of mental disorders can be implemented, as their efficacy is well documented in general practitioners. The need for specific training is suggested by the results of a recent American study, which showed significant gaps in knowledge of psychiatric aspects of skin diseases by dermatologists.

Clearly, the goal of such training programs is not to turn dermatologists into psychiatrists, but rather to make them more capable to recognize the presence of psychopathological symptoms and to help them feel more comfortable in their relationship with patients that are emotionally suffering.

It is also important to make dermatologists aware that an attitude of interest to the emotional aspects does not just lengthen the duration of the visits, but rather can make the consultation more efficient. Communication training programs to improve doctor-patient relation may also be useful, which is related to patient satisfaction and adhesion to the dermatological treatment.

To increase patient identification with a probable mental disorder, you can also promote the use of questionnaires validated in dermatological patients for the screening of a generic psychiatric morbidity, such as GHQ-12, or for the screening of depressive disorders, like the PHQ-9 or the PC-SAD.

However, considered separately, neither the training programs nor those of screenings can lead to a substantial improvement in clinical outcomes. In general medicine, both the implementation of guidelines and training strategies have shown only limited efficacy in modifying clinical practice and in improving the outcome of psychiatric disorders. Screening itself is also insufficient to improve health outcomes if it does not include a filter phase to give feedback to the Doctor on the probable positives and, above all, to actively support the mental health services.

Therefore, if it is true that dermatologists have a key role in identifying psychiatric comorbidity, it must be recognized that they need support from mental health specialists to manage these patients more effectively. The targeted training and screening programs to increase the recognition of psychiatric disorders in dermatological patients should therefore be accompanied by the development of efficient consultation and connection and by the implementation of programs to improve the quality of care. The promotion of a connecting job may be difficult at first, but experience suggests that things tend to improve once some starting contacts are established and maintained.

A particularly important topic is the role of the dermatologist in the prevention of self-injurious gestures. Some patients who come to the attention of the dermatologist, in fact, are at increased risk of suicide. These are patients with skin diseases for which the literature has documented an association with the suicidal ideation (severe psoriasis, acne, atopic dermatitis) and, in general of the people in whom skin pathology is accompanied by deep emotional suffering, body image alterations, difficulties in intimate relationships and impaired daily activities.

In such patients, especially if in the presence of other known risk factors for suicide (for example, history of attempted suicide, severe mental or physical disorders, alcoholism, unemployment, recent mourning or divorce, access to lethal means), a specific assessment should be carried out. It is good to use a prudent and gradual approach, always maintaining an empathic and non-judgmental attitude.

It can start with a general question about the emotional state, and whether the patient expresses feelings of loss of hope, sadness, or loss of interest in life, continue with a question that investigates feelings of the worthlessness of life or desires of death. If the answer is positive, it is imperative to investigate the presence of suicidal thoughts and plans, and any steps the patient may have already taken in the realization of his own suicide plan.

If the evaluation should highlight an imminent suicide risk (for example, detailed and implicit suicide plans, the use of violent means with high lethal potential, difficulty in controlling the impulses, strong determination to end their existence), the situation requires immediate action, and it cannot be limited to a general referral to the psychiatrist. Rather, an emergency psychiatric assessment will be required, pending of which the patient will be kept under careful observation.

The detailed description of a clinical case reported in the literature can be useful to illustrate the importance of a valid and mutual collaboration between dermatologists and mental health specialists. The case concerns a woman of 58 years, hospitalized in a dermatology department, who complained of purulent skin lesions on the back that had spread to the internal organs. In her story, the problem dated back to 7 years, when she had been hospitalized because of a mosquito bite. She reported having suffered from numerous physicists ailments in previous years, for which she had been treated unsuccessfully by various specialists (for example, endocrinologists, gastroenterologists, gynecologists, urologists).

Physical examination and laboratory tests revealed nothing abnormal, except for a small scar on her back, probably due to intense self-scratching. While the patient was hospitalized in the dermatological department, psychiatric counseling was also performed.

The patient was correctly oriented towards space, time, and people, and her cognitive functions were intact. She appeared communicating, and she also reported numerous family problems (she was separated from her alcoholic husband, but still lived with him because of financial difficulties). He complained of a tingling sensation in the back, probably a proprioceptive hallucination, caused in her opinion by viruses and infected fluids that flowed through her body.

Her sleep was bad since she slept in a sitting position to prevent pus from flowing into her head. The anxiety level was high, while the mood was not altered, and affectivity was appropriate. The patient was not aware of the true nature of her problem, she had stopped working due to health problems, and later she had spent most of her spare time consulting the various specialists.

The psychiatrist diagnosed a somatic delusional disorder and prescribed sulpiride treatment at a dose of 200 mg/day, together with a dermatological treatment consisting of the application of ointment with paraffin and vitamin to improve the general condition of the patient's skin.

Dermatologists justified the psychopharmacological

prescription explaining to the patient the close connections between the nervous system and the skin, including the common origin from the ectoderm, and proposing a "psychosomatic" vision of her condition. After a week, the patient was discharged and referred to the dermatological clinic of the same hospital.

Because of her resistance to being treated by a psychiatrist, the dermatological checkups were scheduled more frequently (every month) than psychiatric ones (every three months) to encourage adherence to the treatment. Six months after discharge from the hospital, the somatic discomforts had slightly eased, and the patient could sleep in a semi-sitting position.

The case illustrates very well the fundamental the importance of an integrated biopsychosocial approach: Doctors who had treated the patient in previous years had failed to send her to a psychiatrist, while the therapeutic strategy to welcome her into the Dermatology Department, and to make her gradually aware of the nature of her condition and role of psychological factors, were successful in the construction and the maintenance of a valid therapeutic alliance.

As for the interventions, the realistic goals of psychiatric comorbidity treatment in dermatological patients are: reduce itching and scratching, improve sleep, reduce psychopathological symptoms such as depression, anxiety, embarrassment, and social withdrawal, increase the sense of personal control, encourage acceptance of the unpleasant aspects of skin pathologies not susceptible to a decisive treatment.

The choice of the psychotropic drug obviously depends on the type of mental disorder. The action profile of tricyclic antidepressant drugs, which includes ant-histaminergic effects, anticholinergic effects, and centrally-mediated analgesic effects, can be useful in many clinic situations that can be found in dermatology. Among non-drug treatments, in addition to psychotherapy, relaxation can also be used in certain cases, meditation, hypnosis, bio-feedback.

For effective treatment of psychiatric comorbidity, it is essential that the dermatologist can make use of a well-functioning consultation and connection service, to ask for counseling and to send at least part of the patients. Therefore, it is essential to build an effective collaboration that respects the mutual competences between dermatologists and mental health specialists.

Psychopharmacological and psychosocial treatments, in addition to the primary objective of reducing psychopathological symptoms, may have the suggestive goal to improve the state of the skin pathology. Randomized controlled trials have provided evidence, albeit only preliminary, that such an effect is possible, at least in some patients with certain dermatological pathologies:

- In a study, the hair regrowth was observed in 5 out of 7 patients with alopecia aerate treated with imipramine, compared to no results in 6 patients treated with placebo;

- In another study of patients with vitiligo, regression of lesions was observed in 3 out of 8 patients treated with a short cycle of 8 cognitive-behavioral psychotherapy sessions, while a worsening of the lesions has been observed in 2 out of 8 patients in the waiting list of the control group.

- In a study out of 37 psoriasis patients treated with phototherapy or photo-chemotherapy, adding a meditation-based stress reduction program, the healing time has significantly reduced.

- In another study on 40 patients with psoriasis treated with phototherapy, an intervention to facilitate the emotional expression through the written summary of stressful experiences has lengthened the duration of remission of lesions after the end of phototherapy.

Here is a summary of the management of the dermatological patient according to a biopsychosocial approach:

- In the collection of the near and remote anamnesis, assess whether the skin pathology is related temporal (current or previous) with a critical phase of the life cycle development (childhood, adolescence) or with a delicate phase of the life cycle of adulthood (e.g., taking a serious person sentimental commitment, transition from middle age, retirement);

- In the clinical evaluation of the severity of the pathology, give particular weight to the more relevant body areas on an emotional level (face, neck, hands, and genital area), bearing in mind that a mild clinical disease can have a strong emotional impact if it causes significant harm on body image for the patient;

- Assess the impact of skin pathology on quality of life, giving particular weight to compromises in the quality of intimate and emotional relationships and to limitations in work activities (for example, works involving contact with the public) or free time (for example, sports that involve the use of clothing that leaves ample uncovered areas such as swimsuit, shorts, tank tops);

- If logistically feasible, associate to the clinical quality of life assessment also a standardized assessment with tool for dermatological conditions (Skindex, DLQI) to be completed in the waiting room;

- Assess the level of emotional stress related to the presence of the pathology and its relationship with the course of the pathology itself;

- Assess the role of other potentially stressful events or situations;

- Do not assume that a patient who is not being followed by a mental health specialist is free of psychiatric comorbidity. Collect news about previous mental disorders and treatment, and carry out a lean psychiatric assessment that includes the basics (form and content of thought, mood, anxiety level, sleep quality, aggressiveness, impulse control ability);

- Assess the feasibility and usefulness of associating a standardized assessment of psychopathology with a validated and agile psychiatric screening questionnaire to be completed in the waiting room;

- In patients whose skin pathology is accompanied by deep emotional pain, changes in body image, difficulties in intimate relationships, and impaired daily activities, especially in the presence of other risk factors for suicide (for example, history of attempted suicide, severe mental or physical ailments, alcoholism, unemployment, recent mourning or divorce, access to firearms or other lethal means), carry out an evaluation of the suicide risk;

- Dedicate clinical attention to all situations in which there is marked emotional distress or a formally diagnosed mental disorder;

- In view of the alliance and trust link between doctor and patient, various patients may take great advantage of simple interventions of the dermatologist (give the patient more information on the pathology, its treatment, and its course; provide support and reassurance; moderate and judicious use of psychotropic drugs according to experience and skills of the dermatologist);

- The dermatologist will be able to send to a mental health specialist all cases he doesn't feel comfortable treating himself.

3.5 Conclusions

Dermatology is one of the fields of medicine in which the mutual links between mind and body stand out with greater force, and the link between mind and skin is covered by a vast literature. Studies show that the psychosocial aspects form an integral part of skin pathologies and that in several dermatological patients, there are complex health needs that are not limited to the skin itself.

The systematic inclusion of psychological aspects and social functioning in the elements of clinical evaluation, combined with the development of a mutual and respectful collaboration between dermatologists and mental health specialists, are the necessary steps to achieve an integrated biopsychosocial approach and improve the clinical outcomes for these patients.

Chapter 4 - Stress and functional gastrointestinal disorders

4.1 Introduction

This chapter takes into consideration the interactions between psychophysical stress and functional gastrointestinal disorders. The latter represent a family of dysfunctional affections with a high prevalence in the general population, causing morbidity and very relevant socio-sanitary costs, even in the presence of good laboratory results or anatomical-morphological tests.

For this reason, the functional gastrointestinal disorders (FGIDs) are often considered virtual disorders, that is, present only in the patient "mind," and therefore are neglected by most gastroenterologists and general practitioners, with the result of keeping a significant symptomatic expression and high suffering in the patient, perpetuating psychological stress, related to the lack of understanding of the disorder itself.

4.2 Functional gastrointestinal disorders

The symptoms related to non-structural or "functional" disorders can sometimes represent a clinical enigma, as they often remain without a clear explanation or effective therapy. These symptoms are adversely affected by being considered, also by experienced clinicians, as related to "minor" problems, greatly amplified from the patient's psychic and socio-cultural factors, even in the presence of good results in the tests. In other words, these are disorders that violate the traditional medical paradigm, in which the doctor searches for the signs and symptoms of a disease (inflammatory, infectious, and neoplastic) to arrive at a diagnosis and offer a specific treatment; in this case, vice versa, the symptoms reported by the patient cannot be explained with this simple linear model, being generated by the complex interaction of biological, psychological and social factors affecting the "normal functioning" of an organ or apparatus.

Even after many years from the historical introduction in Gastroenterology of diagnostic criteria for FGIDs, it should be considered that generally the diagnosis is made by exclusions; in fact, there is no real "culture" of functional disorders or a formal training that makes the specialist capable of their easy diagnosis.

As proof of this, the American Gastroenterological Association has verified that the most frequent expressions of doctors to describe FGIDs are "disorder without structural, infectious or metabolic causes" (the most frequent) or "stress disorder" or "gastrointestinal motility disorder."

It is historically believed that such a culturally negative attitude towards general functional disorders has its roots in the ancient Cartesian separation between mind and body, in which the disease was defined on the basis of the encountered organic alterations. A modern holistic vision, which is also considered in gastroenterology, vice versa, conceives the mind and body as parts of a unique system in which the failure to regulate one of these two components produces discomfort and disease.

Therefore, FGIDs are defined as biopsychosocial disorders related to an alteration or dysregulation of the brain-gut axis, which leads to alterations in the perception of visceral pain, in some autonomic functions, and in central processing of visceral stimuli. This model takes into account, on one hand, the correlation between peripheral (intestinal) factors of the Irritable Bowel Syndrome (IBS) such as motility and intestinal perception, and central factors such as traumatic or stressful experiences, frequently reported by patients; and on the other, the frequent psychiatric comorbidity of patients with IBS, particularly concerning anxiety and depression, and finally luminal factors such as inflammation (in particular, in the case of IBS, with post-infectious genesis), and perhaps also the composition of the intestinal microbiota.

Identify the biological mechanisms of hyper-reactivity to

stress in patients with IBS can be helpful to both identify new drug targets and to encourage an effective treatment approach for the individual patient, to possibly reduce the high social and economic costs of IBS.

Here is a scheme to summarize the biopsychosocial model of functional gastrointestinal disorders (FGIDs) for interpretation of pathogenesis, clinical expression, and outcome. SNC, Central Nervous System; SNE, Enteric Nervous System:

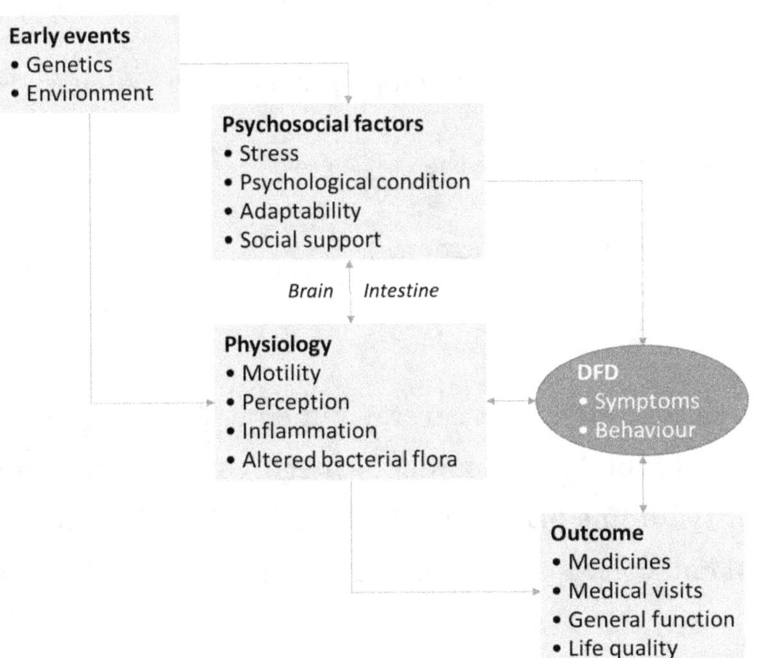

4.3 Classification of Functional gastrointestinal disorders

From the 80s, FGIDs have increasingly been recognized as an autonomous clinical entity from the scientific community, and this represented the true and proper *conditio sine qua non* to arrive at a standardization in the diagnostic criteria of this pathology. FGIDs (in adults) are classified into six overall areas:

1. Esophageal (category A);

2. Gastroduodenal (category B);

3. Intestinal (category C);

4. Functional abdominal pain syndrome (category D);

5. Biliary (category E);

6. Anus-rectal (category F).

Each category includes several ailments. For example, the intestinal functional disorders (category C) include irritable bowel syndrome (IBS) (C1), the functional swelling (C2), the functional constipation (C3), and the functional diarrhea (C4).

Although some symptoms (pain, bloating, diarrhea, and constipation) may be present in more disorders, IBS, for example, is more specifically defined as pain or abdominal discomfort associated with changes in the belly.

In this chapter, we will mainly deal with IBS, as regards the interactions between stress and FGIDs. The pathogenesis of this syndrome sees a combination of various factors, from genetics to alteration of intestinal motility, of visceral sensitivity, immune regulation at the level of the mucosa, to changes in bacterial flora, and finally to the alteration of the regulation between the enteric system and the central nervous (brain-gut axis).

The interaction between these factors is their relative contribution can vary greatly from patient to patient and also in the same patient in later times, consequently generating the need for clinical approaches and therapeutic programs aimed at the specific conditions.

4.4 Stress and FGIDs

Stressors can have an acute or chronic effect and a range that varies from daily events to situations that could potentially compromise the survival itself, such as natural disasters, physical or psychological violence. The reals stressors are capable of activating adaptive responses of the "fight or flight" type.

Over time, chronic or recurrent stress involves a

commitment to the various physiological systems that have to face it, defined as "allostatic load," which can lead to behavioral changes, physiological reactivity, or biological alterations for the whole organism that can lead to even significant ailments. The anti-stress or allostatic systems primarily include the hypothalamic-pituitary-adrenal axis, then the autonomic and immune nervous systems, and finally, the cardio-vascular and metabolic one.

Excessive allostatic load occurs clinically with fatigue, irritability, sense of demoralization along with various other visceral and somatic symptoms, often reported by patients with IBS and other FGIDs. A large number of evidences supports the role of stress in the pathophysiology of IBS. The conceptual model related to the effect of stress in the patient with IBS assumes that, in the genetically predisposed subject, chronic stress can determine a response persistently increased on central stress circuits and a facilitation of the development of functional and affective disorders.

In particular, the effect of stress in IBS is to modify the normal interaction of the brain-gut axis, a set of hierarchically organized homeostatic reflexes, starting from neuronal circuits contained in the enteric nervous system and gradually converging towards the spinal cord, the midbrain, the hypothalamic structures, and amygdala, up to the insular cortex and anterior cingulate.

4.5 Association with early stressful events

Early stressful events (ESE) are traumatic experiences during childhood, represented, for example, by a maladaptive relationship with a parent or caregiver, a serious illness, the death of a parent, or sexual abuse.

Various studies suggest that ESEs cause major brain dysfunction, which mainly consists of an alteration of the homeostasis of the neurobiological systems' response to stress, which leads to an increase in vulnerability towards long-term behavioral and social disturbances.

In this context, there are scientific evidences that stress and, in particular, sexual abuse can also influence the clinical outcome, causing more troublesome symptoms, a higher frequency of specialist visits, and a worse performance in work or personal activities of the patients.

A paradigmatic ESE is the one related to sexual abuse, physical and/or emotional, in particular, if it occurred in childhood. In IBS, the percentages of individuals with positive results of sexual abuse range from 30 to 56%, depending on the disorder and on the reference specialist center.

The percentages of patients with a history of abuse are significantly greater than both healthy individuals and patients with organic gastroenterological disorders. Interestingly, only 17% of abused victims had talked to their doctor about it, and about 30% had never told anyone about it. These figures suggest that, despite the enormous emotional impact and its important repercussions on health and quality of life, this trauma remains essentially hidden in many cases.

A history of abuse involves more severe symptoms and poor therapeutic results in many cases of IBS, as also derived from the observation that the prevalence of abuse in patients with mild IBS is about a third lower than the one observed in patients with severe IBS. In addition, patients with a history of sexual abuse suffer more frequently than others of concomitant symptoms such as anxiety disorders, depressive symptoms, panic attacks, chronic fatigue, insomnia, headache, pelvic pain.

Again, it has been reported a sort of "dose effect" in the sense that the victims of serious abuse such as rape or physical abuse that endangered life, present a compromised healthier state compared to subjects with a history of less serious abuse. It seems finally proved that previous abuse and the DFD status contribute independently to compromise the quality of life.

A pathophysiological link between sexual abuse and changes in the central nervous system as a consequence of stress was identified using sophisticated investigations like magnetic resonance imaging (MRI): these studies show that in IBS patients, during pneumatic rectal distension, a greater activation of the anterior and posterior cingulate cortex is observed, with respect to subjects of control.

It has been speculated that such activation could be a biological marker of a state of chronic pain and/or psychological stress. Interesting is the preliminary data that the activation of this cortical area can be reduced with a clinical-induced improvement by psychopharmacological or cognitive-behavioral therapy: however, further studies are needed to confirm these data.

4.6 Psychophysical stress and post-infectious IBS

The importance of chronic stress in compromising the clinical outcome causing more annoying symptoms, more frequent specialist visits, and a worse quality of life has also been recognized in the clinical variant of IBS termed Post-Infectious (IBS-PI), which originates after an acute episode of acute gastroenteritis which apparently does not resolve itself but tends to become chronic. In an older study, it has been verified that chronic stress and some psychological characteristics such as hypochondria can predict the incidence of IBS-PI regardless of age, gender, and social status.

The scheme of the stress response system is summarized below. The action of the Hypothalamic-Pituitary-Adrenal axis (HPA) in stress response is well known. Neurons in the medial parvocellular region of the hypothalamus release CRH and Arginine-Vasopressin (AVP) that determines the secretion of ACTH (Adreno Cortico Tropic Hormone) from the pituitary gland, with the production of glucocorticoids from the adrenal gland.

The stress-induced HPA answer is modulated by feedback between glucocorticoids, ACTH, and CRF. Under normal conditions, after the activation of the HPA system and the cessation of the stressful event, there is a feedback mechanism that disables the HPA response. The amygdala can vice versa maintain the effect on the HPA axis if the stressful condition persists, while the hippocampus has an inhibitory action.

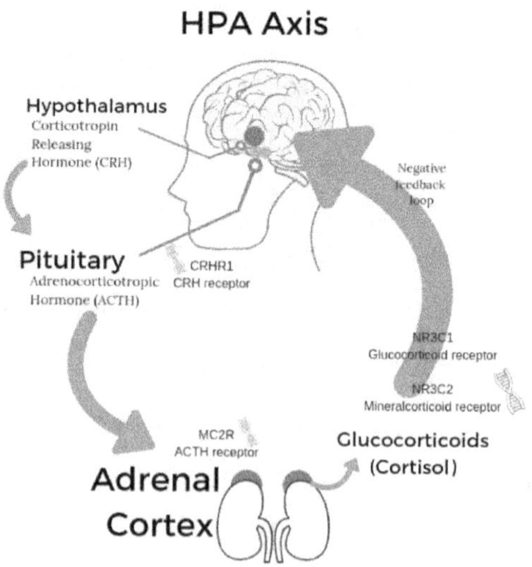

4.7 Bidirectional gut-brain relationships (role of the CRF)

The relationship between stressful events and the gastrointestinal system can be viewed as a direct consequence of the bidirectional modulation of the gastrointestinal function by the central nervous system, which includes motor responses, pain modulation, and also immune functions.

According to more modern neurological researches, neurobiological changes induced by stress occur both in central circuits and in arousal mechanisms of the emotional circuit; these outputs concern the parasympathetic and sympathetic nervous system, the Hypothalamic-Pituitary-Adrenal (HPA) axis, the endogenous modulation systems of pain and the neuro-transmitter ascending pathways.

Various stressors are able to activate these output systems, involving some somatic functions and also the patient's behavior. Both neuropsychological responses (in particular anxiety, hypervigilance, and arousal) and hormonal changes induced by stress are strongly linked to the increase of the release of Corticotropin Releasing Factor (CRF), a hypothalamic neuro-hormone which activates the HPA axis and the autonomic nervous system, which then activate some noradrenergic routes, such as the noradrenergic of the locus coeruleus system.

The release of CRF from the paraventricular nucleus of the hypothalamus is under the excitatory control of the central nuclei of the amygdala and hippocampal inhibitor.

The way of CRF is also able to stimulate anxiety and visceral responsiveness regardless of the HPA axis. The expression of the CRF and the two receptors so far identified (CRF1 and CRF2), which are part of the G-protein-coupled receptor family, appears tissue-specific, dependent on physiological conditions, and influenced by environmental stimuli.

However, most studies on the CRF pathway are still based on an animal model, where CRF1 receptor antagonists have been shown to be able to counteract hypervigilance or anxiety behaviors, to diminish automatic dysfunctions, and at the same time, to counteract the increase in colic motility, in the increased permeability of the colic mucosa, in the activation of mast cells (related to abdominal pain) and in hypersensitivity to colorectal distension, precisely those changes present in many IBS patients.

Studies on humans are still initial, although preliminary data are coming from a phase 1 randomized controlled clinical trial indicate that an antagonist of CRF1 (the NBI-34041) can attenuate the neuroendocrine response to psychosocial stress of male control subjects. Other studies have tested the efficacy of CRF1 antagonists in anxiety-depressive situations, but they have reported mixed results. An interesting fact is that many psychotropic drugs, including tricyclic antidepressants, are able to reduce CRF levels.

Such drugs are commonly used in the therapy of patients with IBS and dominant diarrhea (IBS-D); this data seems to indicate that an alteration of the pathway of the CRF can be an important mechanism that influences pain perception and other IBS symptoms. In fact, in the experimental animal, activation of central and peripheral CRF1 receptors potentiates the motor response and colon secretory, with the development of diarrhea.

It is very likely that the stress-induced CRF activation happens from the center to the periphery: in fact, psychological stressors are able to activate the CRF system initially in the brain, with the induction of alterations of the colic function related to the autonomic nervous system.

Autonomic alterations are then able to stimulate the CRF system in the colon, as part of this response, and thus create the whole intestinal symptoms. The mechanisms of autonomic alterations include an increase in colic serotonin that is active on 5-HT3 and 5-HT4 receptors, mediated by cholinergic parasympathetic activation. This has been proven experimentally and also in humans using 5-HT3 antagonists such as the granisetron and ondansetron.

The CRF is, therefore, a ubiquitous and essential mediator in the dynamics of the brain-gut axis. It should be reiterated that the interaction between the brain and the enteric system is bidirectional, and it is now proven that a dysfunction of one of the two extremes immediately affects the other.

4.8 Stress-induced changes in intestinal functions

On an experimental level, it is known that stress induces diffuse motor alterations on a gastrointestinal level. Over 20 years ago, scholars have shown, for example, that IBS patients have an increase in colic motor activity at rest and that the response to stress experimental physical or psychological stress compared to healthy control individuals is much greater.

Other studies have shown stress-induced motor alterations also in intestinal districts other than the colon (gastric antrum and small intestine), which supports the concept of an effect of the stress on the entire gastrointestinal motility in patients with IBS.

For what it concerns visceral perception, experimental studies conducted in patients with IBS have shown that stress is able to increase it; for example, some studies suggest different behavior in healthy subjects and in patients with IBS during psychological stress and simultaneous painless rectal stimulation: the former show a significant increase in the sensory threshold (reduced perception), while no change is observed in the latter.

Also, in patients with IBS stimulated after the conclusion of psychological stress, a significant reduction of the sensory threshold (increased perception) was observed, while in the control people this was not observed. Finally, IBS patients reported a score of psychological stress higher than controls during the rectal distension course.

Very similar data come from other studies where psychological stress was represented by an auditory stimulus, and the visceral stimulation was still impacting the pneumatic phasic distension of the rectum, obtained with a balloon inflated up to a pressure of 45 mmHg, or by an electric current on the mucous membrane of the rectum and the physical stress was represented by the immersion in the cold water of the non-dominant hand, alternating with a psychological stimulus (dichotomous listening).

All these studies support the notion that subjects with IBS have a reduction in the visceral perception threshold, an alteration that some years ago, it was indicated as the biological marker of IBS itself.

Less clear are the changes induced by stress on intestinal secretion and permeability; the latter appears to have increased in patients with IBS and dominant diarrhea (IBS-D) compared with control patients. Also, for this alteration, it seems proven, so far in the animals only, that CRF plays an important role.

As for secretion, there is a recent study conducted on young women with IBS, which showed how physical stress represented by immersion in the cold water of the hand, associate with a modification of the intestinal water outflow, and with an increase in the output of chlorides and albumin from fasting, suggesting that (acute) stress may affect intestinal secretion.

4.9 Conclusions

From the above data, which in particular refer to IBS that seems to be the more frequent of the DFD, this pathology can be considered to be strongly influenced by stress (stress-sensitive disorder). In a predisposed subject, chronic stress can induce an increased response of the central stress circuits, a dysregulation of the adaptive systems, and finally, a particular propensity towards abdominal symptoms.

In this scenario, early stressful events play a decisive role, since they invariably accompany pathological disease behaviors and multiple functional pathologies. Animal models and, in part, human studies have also documented how much early psychophysical stress impacts the development of IBS and on a persistent tendency to over-respond to chronic stress, probably mediated by mechanisms in which CRF appears to be the main actor.

Finally, chronic stress certainly has a negative impact on the clinical outcome and natural history of IBS. If it is clear that both factors, the peripheral and central ones, can trigger the symptoms, it is certainly their continuous interaction in the brain-intestine axis that perpetuates the stress-induced alterations of the gastrointestinal function, of the autonomic and neuroendocrine responses, and of the pain modulation.

The conclusion is that early identification of stress-induced symptoms may allow for more effective management of IBS, for example, by introducing treatments for stress management and cognitive-behavioral therapies that can probably contribute to reducing the high social and economic costs.

Chapter 5 - Stress and immune system

Research over the past few decades has been able to offer data that has enabled to overcome a pure scientific vision of the organism:

a. Fragmented, i.e., based on the idea of relatively autonomous or biological systems in their functions and reduced reciprocal communications;

b. Deterministic, based on the genetics "central dogma," which sees the phenotype as a linear implementation of the genotype, and not related to environmental and experiential influences;

c. Dualistic, i.e., set to a substantial separation between mind and body.

To understand human functioning, we need data on the following levels of functions, seen as interdependent:

- Psychological and behavioral (states and traits);

- Brain;

- Information transfer systems (autonomic, endocrine

nervous system, immune);

- Properties of the organism (functions of organs and peripheral physiology).

There is recognition of the fact that all living matter is organized and presents itself as structured within networks (biological systems are made up of multilevel networks: proteins, genomics, cellular, etc.), which can be studied in their static and dynamic properties, allowing you to open new horizons of research but also new therapies.

The peculiar ability of the brain to work in parallel and on several subjects in parallel allows this organ (which expresses the highest biological complexity known today) to manage the connections between the psychic aspect of life and the somatic aspect, especially through information transfer systems: nervous system autonomous, endocrine and immune.

This communications network modulates and holds together the whole body network, which also has rules, needs, and own specificities that continually feedback with the brain-mind system. It should not be forgotten that, unlike a machine (which becomes a whole starting from single and separate "pieces"), the living being articulates its elements starting from a unity, and such unitary character is in every small part of the biological organism.

Many areas of study have contributed to this result, typically interdisciplinary research areas such as the stress or what is defined as "psycho-neuro-endocrine immunology" (PNEI). Studies on stress have shown the role of this fundamental physiological mechanism (able to enlist and modify all biological systems, in the short and in the long period) and its constant action in modulating subjective behaviors aimed at any type of adaptation (species-specific and individual-specific).

On the other hand, PNEI has allowed us to frame not only the integration of the different systems but also between the central regulatory processes and peripheral physiology.

5.1 Brain, endocrine, and immune system

The "history" of PNEI began in the 60s when it was demonstrated for the first time how learnings can act on immune activity (by activating, increasing, or decreasing it). This data involved the connection between the central nervous system (CNS) and immunity, and the relationship - via the brain - between mental input and immune activity. In the following years, the physiological foundations of these interactions began to be highlighted.

In the 80s, researchers discovered a network of nerves that unites blood vessels and cells of the immune system, and nerves are also discovered in the thymus and spleen with terminations near lymphocyte and macrophage heap. A decisive step was taken after the discovery that immune cells can produce the same type of hormones produced by the brain (neuropeptides) and how this allows bidirectional communication.

Scholars speculated that the immune system also serves as a "fluid sense organ" for stimuli from bacteria and viruses, and as such, represents the connection with the brain to coordinate the organism response. This function explains the connection between the nervous, endocrine, and immune systems, which act as a large integrated network.

The life of each being is guaranteed by its ability to attribute meaning and to react accordingly to stimuli produced by the environment or by its own actions: we can divide these stimuli into cognitive and non-cognitive. The former are tried using the neuroendocrine system and are generally taken to some mental-processing level; for the non-cognitive ones (allergens, viruses, bacteria, etc.), it is instead the immune system that has the task of processing and informing the body.

An adequate response requires the integration of this information: this helps to understand why antigens and psychic stimuli evoke an integrated immune-neuroendocrine response, basically similar, and also because some constant correlations between the integrity of the individual psychic structure and the integrity of the immune activity have emerged.

The three systems, through communication and mutual regulation processes, play, in dynamic balance, the role of health balance, thanks to the dialogue of the common mediators (neurotransmitters, hormones, peptides) that bind to receptors of the target cells, stimulating or repressing the cellular response.

Both nervous system and immune system have in common, in addition to stimuli perception, the learning ability, the memory (neural memory and immune memory), and the mediators (molecules) that act on the three systems.

5.1.1 Stress, adaptation and health

In this context, a strategic role is played by the stress circuits. It's about processes developed by evolution to manage and distribute energy in relation to the need for adaptation of the individual. Stress is an attempt to maintain a balance by eliminating or reducing a discrepancy.

The brain-mind system, in relation to hereditary and experiential parameters (and therefore with a significant variability and an individual specificity), identifies the situations that determine a gap in the adaptive balances (physiological, psychological, and social), and which are therefore threatening for the individual.

The brain structures that support these processes include the hippocampus, the amygdala, and areas of the prefrontal cortex, which activate a neuroendocrine circuit (HPA - Hypothalamus-Pituitary-Adrenal) and a circuit based on the peripheral nervous system, able to activate the physiological and psycho-behavioral response of the individual.

The limbic system in bidirectional integration with the cortices (in particular prefrontal) supports emotions and cognition that are activities that assign meanings and emotional tone to external and internal stimuli, using both implicit and explicit memory circuits for this purpose (emotional and cognitive information processing).

Through these structures, the brain-mind system modulates the activation of the biological devices, whose activity feeds back on the brain and on the mind itself. The hypothalamus, located between the centers of the base of the brain, is the common activator structure of the stress circuits.

It is considered as the interface between the mental and the physiology-vegetative levels because, with its connections and functions, it integrates stimuli from higher centers and information from peripheral organs and from the body, and translates these changes into variations in physiological parameters and in the execution of innate basic behavioral patterns related to survival and to reproduction. The neurons of the paraventricular nuclei of the hypothalamus, when are called to do so, release two substances, CRH or CRF (hormone or factor of corticotropin release) and AVP (arginine-vasopressin).

These substances together induce the pituitary to produce the Adreno Cortico Tropic Hormone (ACTH), which through the bloodstream, stimulates the bark of the adrenal glands producing glucorticolids, including cortisol.

The pituitary, also called "pituitary gland," is the most important hormone-regulating structure and a strategic link between the nervous and endocrine systems. The substances produced by the pituitary are fundamental in the regulation of many activities (metabolism, fluid regulation, reproduction and sexuality, growth, and so on), both by direct action or by action on other glands, such as the thyroid.

The action of glucocorticoids (cortisol in humans) is to produce a general mobilization of the organism's resources. The action of cortisol takes place by modulating the metabolism (increased production of glucose in the liver, increased mobilization of free fatty acids by making more energy available for combustion, increased availability of glucose in the brain, stimulation of the use of proteins for energy production), and stimulating reactions of the immune system.

The other way, the "nervous" one, is always activated by the hypothalamus, which sends signals to some nerve structures located in the brain stem, in particular in the locus coeruleus, with the release of norepinephrine that goes towards the brain and with activation of the sympathetic nervous system towards the rest of the body (internal organs, blood vessels, skin).

The sympathetic fibers from the spinal cord with a very direct route (i.e., without intermediate synapses) reach the medullary portion of the adrenal glands (which is located inside the adrenals), where the production of a mixture of exciting substances is stimulated, collectively called catecholamine, largely composed of adrenaline and, to a lesser extent, from norepinephrine and dopamine.

Catecholamine affects the function of various organs: increase the cardiac activity, both the pressure and the blood flow, diverting the flow of blood to the muscles and kidneys, reducing the diameter of the blood vessels in the periphery and increasing it in the liver and muscles.

The so-called "autonomous" nervous system responds quickly to stress, and it controls the activity of many organs and systems of the human body, such as the cardiovascular, respiratory, gastrointestinal, renal, and endocrine. The two ways, the neuroendocrine and the SNA one, are intertwined, with numerous points of interaction.

For example, the neurons that produce CRH (Corticotropin-Releasing Hormone) are in connection with those who produce norepinephrine in the locus coeruleus, and they influence each other reciprocally.

Bidirectional stress processes are protective for the individual, and they promote the adaptation (allostasis). However, the excessive or dysfunctional use of these processes can cause conditions of progressive dysregulation, which determines a state of physical and mental malaise that compromises resilience and health.

Researches on stress have focused on several aspects, in relation to prevailing approaches and interests:

- On the stress "sources" (environment, stimuli), where a sociological vision prevails;

- On the consequences (reaction, malaise, illness), marked by a psychosomatic and biomedical vision;

- On subjective evaluation processes, basically thorough in the psychological field.

Nowadays it seems necessary to integrate these aspects into an approach that could be defined as PNEI or biopsychosocial, capable of synthesizing the systemic role of these processes in relation to life and health of the person in relation to its history and current context.

The "Stress Libra model" was presented as a contribution in this area of discussion, where stress is the product of the self-regulatory balance between the individual and context and between requests and resources.

From the meeting of these dimensions, four factors (external requests, internal requests, internal resources, and resources external) are highlighted, which determine - in their mutual interaction - the quantitative and qualitative levels of both physiological and psychological stress.

5.1.2 Stress and immunity

PNEI research has shown how stress induces changes in the immune activity, that there are relationships between immunity, psychological distress, and personality, and finally, that our immune "competence" is modular].

The interaction between the Central Nervous System (CNS) and the Immune System (IS) occurs at many levels, via neurotransmitters, cytokines, and hormones. The main link is represented by the hypothalamic-pituitary-adrenal axis, by the autonomous nervous system (ANS) (sympathetic, noradrenergic, and parasympathetic cholinergic), and by the peptide network, non-cholinergic and non-adrenergic.

The main peptides in this network are the vasoactive intestinal peptides (VIP, Vasoactive Intestinal Peptide), the substance P (SP), and the peptide linked to the calcitonin gene (CGRP, Calcitonin Gene-Related Peptide).

ANS, as is known, innervates important SI-related organs and systems, such as the spleen, liver, thymus, spinal cord, lymph nodes, skin, digestive tract, and respiratory system.

The brain modulates immune activity by neurotransmitters (acetylcholine, noradrelin, setoronin, histamine, glutamate, gamma-aminobutyric acid or gamma-GABA), neuropeptides (adrenocorticotropic hormone or ACTH, prolactin, vasopressin, somatostatin, VIP, SP, neuropeptide Y, encephalins, endorphins), growth factors (neuronal growth factors or NGF, Neuronal Growth Factors) and hormones (adrenaline and glucocorticoids). The SI modulates nerve cells by means of cytokines and chemokines.

Many immune cells have neurotransmitter receptors, neuropeptides, and hormones, and their behavior can be directly influenced through the receptors or indirectly as a result of the action of the cytokines, following CNS activation.

The action of stress on the SI is quite complex and testifies to the stress adaptive value. Immune modulation seems to be linked precisely to the nature of the stressful experience for the individual. The literature has highlighted apparently discordant data which we have tried to explain, taking into account how evolution may have selected different response profiles to different stresses in the different species and different immune functions in relation to the physiological response of the body. Thus these apparently discordant results can be understood in different animal species and stressful situations, in vitro and in vivo.

The nature of the stressful situation determines the type of immune responses in different ways, which deal with the parameters of the stressful stimulus (intensity, duration, nature) and with the physiological implications of the same, which involve different immune response profiles.

Innate (genetic) and acquired (experiences) factors, which are interdependent, determine individual differences in stress levels, influencing evaluation processes, the consequent physiological responses, as well as the strategies of overcoming: They determine, therefore, beyond the objective data of the initial stimulus, the intensity, and duration of the stress itself.

It is evolutionarily understandable that a threatening situation (aggression or accident) triggers an acute process of stress and accompanies an immune activation (injury and infection) and which, in turn, many situations involving an immune activation can stimulate stress-related processes. The acute stress understood as a short-term experience (from minutes to hours), translates into a condition that requires the mobilization of the body's defenses, including the immune ones.

Although in man, as is known, this process can be triggered from psychological stimuli (relational, social, internal experiences, etc.), the consequent physiological process is evolutionarily calibrated on an archaic "attack-escape" response with a high probability of physical aggression and, therefore, of immune protection.

Immune activation is therefore consistent with the short term physiological response to stress, because it translates into a condition of "immuno-protection" from potential (real or imaginary) dangers, which physiologically is analogous to what the body activates with situations, such as vaccinations or injuries, involving the need for immune defense.

It is intuitive that this condition if prolonged over time, can cause negative effects, and in fact it has been observed how a situation of protracted stress can reduce and depress the immune response, and as a chronicization of activation from stress (chronic stress) go to dysregulate the immune responses by altering the balance of cytokines, accelerating immune-senescence, suppressing immunity by reducing the number and activities of protective immune cells and an increase in regulatory-inhibitory T cells.

To understand the different relationships of immune components with experience of stress, some authors have proposed to group the different types of innate and acquired or adaptive responses in relation to their situations, so in relationship with the final produced effect. Thus, we speak of "protective immunity," "pathological," and "regulatory-inhibitory" in order to conceptualize models that consider different contributions and behavior (especially in vivo) of the various components of the immune response.

In this context, the actions that promote wound healing can be considered immune-protective, repair of tissues, the elimination of infections or carcinogens, and the induced memory from vaccines. Innate immunity and acquired immunity, both type 1 and type 2, contribute to this. "Pathogenic" immunity is directed against the "self" (autoimmune diseases) or against harmless antigens (asthma, allergies), and which causes states of chronic inflammation.

Finally, responses produced by immune cells and factors that inhibit or suppress the functions of other immune cells are defined as "regulatory-inhibitory": this includes regulatory T lymphocytes CD4+ CD25+ FoxP3+, interelukin10 (IL-10), and the Beta transforming growth factor (TGF), with the aim of keeping under control the pro-inflammatory, the allergic and the autoimmune answers.

5.1.3 Conclusions

Before moving on to treat more closely some pathologies of the immune or immuno-mediated system that arise from a stressful condition, we can summarize as follows:

- The human body is a highly integrated reality aimed at establishing adaptive balances in the surrounding world. The ability to achieve these adaptations vary from individual to individual in relation to innate and acquired interdependent factors;

- Stress represents the energy activated to achieve these adaptations, and this explains the intersubjective variability between objective conditions and levels of psychological and physiological stress;

- The mind-biological systems network, mediated by the interconnections between nervous, endocrine, and immune systems, shows its ability to change psychophysiological and behavioral conditions through the stress circuits. Intensity and duration of stress determine its short or long-term effects on the organism;

- What happens at the immune level is coherent, from an evolutionary point of view, with the role and function of stress, showing immune enhancement as

the first response to stress and a suppressive or
deregulatory tendency with the continuation of the
situation, which increases the susceptibility to the
pathology or, in many cases, actively contributes to
its appearance.

5.2 The pathological consequences of stress on immunity

5.2.1 The dynamics of the immune system

The immune system can activate two different defense
lines, which are strictly connected, and interdependent in a
highly bidirectional way, even if not necessarily, they
always work together.

A first line, entrusted to ancient cells, from the phylogenetic
point of view, which do not abandon us even in old age
when the system declines overall: these are cells capable of
swallowing pathogens, as well as "garbage" that is
generated in the body, internal debris. This mechanism,
called phagocytosis, is mainly carried out by macrophages
and neutrophils.

Phagocytosis is favored by the complement system, a set of
soluble proteins present in the blood, the activation of
which closely resembles the complex mechanisms of

coagulation: these proteins are fixed to the bacterium wall, "marking" it, so favoring its phagocytosis.

Still on the front line, we then find other cells capable of destroying in a rapid way, and without too many "ceremonies" both cells infected by virus and cells transformed in a malicious sense: they are the natural killers (NK). In their front line work, phagocytes and natural killers are helped by other cells: eosinophils, basophils, and mastoids cells, whose role is central to the amplification of the inflammatory response.

This first line of system activation, also called "natural immunity" or innate or non-specific, it can also run out in itself. This is what normally happens in our body, even in situations of limited emergency, when, for example, we need to repair a minor wound, or when we breath, in "moderate" quantity, pathogenic or polluting.

In this regard, it has been calculated that macrophages contained in our pulmonary alveoli can "take care on their own," enduring a bacterial load of up to 1 billion units. Beyond this limit they will call reinforces, releasing signals (cytokines) that will attract dendritic cells, which will activate the lymphocytes.

In cases like these, therefore, the activation of natural immunity entails the consequent activation of the second line, centered on lymphocytes, T and B, called immunity-specific or adaptive or clonotypic.

Recently it was discovered that a family of receptors, called Toll-Like Receptors (TLR), play a fundamental role as a hinge between the two faces of the immunity. TLRs are mounted on different types of natural immunity cells: from macrophages to granulocytes up to dendritic cells.

The dendritic cells that are able to capture the antigen, in a first phase engulf it (as does a macrophage, their close relative) and, subsequently, inside the lymph nodes where they migrated, expose fragments on the surface in front of the lymphocytes.

Lymphocytes are activated in the lymph nodes. Crucial is here the role of T helper (CD4) lymphocytes which, based on the type of antigen presented and on the cytokine profile characterizing the environment in which they operate, and starting from a class of undifferentiated cells (Th naive), can differentiate into regulators Th1, Th2, Th17, and T. So they can give rise to:

1. A response oriented in the cytotoxic sense, with the activation of cytotoxic T lymphocytes (Th1 answer): this answer is supported by INF gamma and IL-12 and is essential against viruses and tumors;

2. An antibody-oriented response, with the activation of B lymphocytes (Th2 type response): this response is supported by IL-4 and IL-13, and it is essential

against bacteria and extracellular parasites;

3. A tolerant response, with the appearance of different types of regulatory T lymphocytes: this response is supported by the IL-10 and TGF Beta and is essential for inflammation control;

4. A prolonged inflammatory response, centered on neutrophils and other cells of natural immunity, with the activation of a T lymphocytes class called Th17: this response is supported by IL-6, IL-23, and IL-17 and it is at the origin of many autoimmune diseases and may also support the same metastatic dissemination of cancer.

But what is influencing the dynamics of the immune system? It is now more and more clear that the different response patterns of the immune system do not depend only from the type of stimulus (a virus, a bacterium, an extracellular parasite, a toxin, a transformed cell), but also from the microenvironment where this meeting with the pathogen takes place, and from the general conditions of the organism and therefore also by psychic stress.

For example, an immune response that occurs within the intestinal or respiratory mucosa will favor the Th2 set with the activation of B lymphocytes and the production of immunoglobulins, first of all, secretory IgA. This answer will circulate lymphocytes that will tend to "join" (homing) in the vast system of mucous membranes (intestinal, respiratory, and urogenital).

Together with the mucous membranes, there are at least two other organs which structurally tend to produce a Th2 response type: the brain and the eye. Both tend to suppress the Th1 and Th17 response type, favoring Th2. Th1 answer is preferably avoided in the mucous membranes, in the eye, and in the brain, because it could produce damages to the tissues themselves: Crohn's disease for the intestine, multiple sclerosis for the nervous system, and uveitis for the eye are included in the context of Th1-Th17 autoimmune diseases. On the contrary, immune activation in the skin, in the blood, in the peripheral lymph nodes will favor the Th1 set with the circulation of cytotoxic T lymphocytes.

Basically, it can be concluded that there is not any correct immune response in itself, but its correctness depends on the place where it is realized and on the predominant type of report it presents. The corollary of this conclusion might sound like this: immune regulation is everything, while the stimulus is nothing. More precisely: the regulation of the response immune is central, while important, but secondary, is the nature of the stimulus that gives rise to the response.

As we have already clarified in the initial part of this

chapter, the psychic stress of chronic type is a powerful factor in altering the dynamics of the immune system, causing suppression and/or dysregulation of the immune response that can be at the origin of numerous and important diseases in which the immune system plays a central role. In the next paragraph are reported some examples without pretending to be comprehensive compared to all possible cases.

5.2.2 Stress and pathologies from immune surveillance failure: infectious diseases and cancer

The psychic stress of chronic type, also as a consequence of trauma in the early stages of life, with dysregulation in the production of cortisol and catecholamine, determines an activation of the Th2 circuit, with the production of inflammatory cytokines typical of this immune profile (IL-4, IL-5, IL-13) and that of the Th17 circuit (IL-17, IL-23).

This type of immune response is unsuitable for fighting viral infections and neoplastic transformed cells, which instead require a Th1 type response. Among the most studied infectious diseases, we include influenza virus infections, herpetic, and acquired immunodeficiency virus.

5.2.2.1 Negative emotions and effectiveness of the flu vaccine

The effectiveness of the flu vaccine is limited and variable: in case of mutations even if apparently not relevant to the viral strain on which the vaccine was built to reduce its effectiveness. But the conditions of the person's immune system who receives the vaccination are also important, which is a real therapeutic immune-induced response.

On "Proceedings of National Academy of Sciences," a group from the University of Wisconsin demonstrated several years ago that a negative psychological state is related to a worse response to the vaccine: so those who are more anxious and depressed produce fewer anti-influenza antibodies.

This result, even if really relevant, is not absolutely new, but it is a confirmation of studies conducted in the 90s of the last century in the field of psycho-neuro-immunological research. Immunologist and psychiatrist from the University of Ohio demonstrated that people dedicated to assisting family members with Alzheimer's responded worse to the flu compared to others.

Now we want to emphasize an important novelty that emerged from the study of other groups, as this research, for the first time, also sought to identify the nerve pathways that produce an immune deficit. The 52 volunteers, between 57 and 60 years old, who in the beginning

December had received the flu shot, they underwent a sophisticated set of psychological tests and electroencephalographic measurements.

People with a more negative emotional style also showed greater activation of the right side of the brain, in particular of the prefrontal cortices; at the same time, they showed an exaggerated response to stimuli given to scare (for example, a loud, sudden sound). In the blood of these people, drawn a few weeks after vaccination, there was a lower antibody titer towards the flu virus than that found in the tubes of their colleagues with a better mood.

 Therefore, the same vaccine produced different results, depending on the emotional state of participants. The link between hyper-activation of the right prefrontal cortices and weakening of the immune response is the subject of a rich scientific literature, which is based on both experimental lesions on animals, and on the less bloody study, on humans with brain damage or even on small children.

For example, in six-month-old babies, it has been shown that greater activation of the right hemisphere is accompanied by an increase of cortisol both under basic conditions and under stimulation.

The hyper-activation of the right prefrontal cortex therefore leads to activation of the stress axis with cortisol overproduction and consequent suppression of the immune response to viruses, namely the Th1 circuit in favor of the ineffective inflammatory Th2 circuit.

5.2.2.2 Stress and herpes

It is known that the herpes simplex virus (HSV) has the ability to remain latent in sensory nerve ganglia and reactivate under stress. Studies of the last fifteen years show that stress not only increases diffusion and severity of herpetic infection in both the peripheral and central nervous systems, but it is also able to suppress the activity of cytotoxic memory T lymphocytes.

Stress disorganizes the immune system circuit that could liquidate or control herpes infection. In addition, a number of studies on animals infected with the virus show that it does reactivates the infection. Finally, studies on women with recurrent or genital herpes on some elderly with shingles (caused by the reactivation of the varicella zoster virus - VZV) demonstrate the same relationship.

In this regard, it is interesting to report that controlled studies demonstrate the effectiveness of ancient techniques for stress management (such as Tai Chi Chuan) in boosting immune control on the varicella-zoster virus in older people undergoing training, compared to the control people involved in the same test.

5.2.2.3 Stress and evolution of HIV infection

Studies of men with HIV infection have shown that stress increases the disease progression, so it speeds up the appearance of AIDS. For example, a prospective study assessed the progress of the disease after 5 and a half years from the beginning, characterized by a complete absence of symptoms.

Patients with higher levels of stress and/or with less social support have developed AIDS three times more frequently than those who had better stress control and/or increased social support. Similarly, other research has reported that homosexual males who tend to hide their sexual identity have an acceleration of the disease.

Finally, studies on the social animals closest to us (the macaques) should be reported, which fall ill with a disease very similar to AIDS caused by a similar virus to HIV, named SIV. They are cruel studies that show, in a shocking way, how much stress counts in the evolution of the disease.

Animals to which the SIV was inoculated, who lived in a stable social environment, had virus concentrations much lower than other macaques that had received the same virus but lived in unstable conditions (for example, the reference group changed every day). And this obviously reflected on the progress of the disease.

The former, socially stable and therefore with less stress, lived longer than their peers forced into an unstable and stressed life. Same virus, same experimental conditions, only varying the stability of the environment of life. And this is precisely what determines the course of the disease.

5.2.2.4 Stress, immunity and cancer

Cancer is a disease that can depend on several factors, and its genesis (carcinogenesis) goes through multiple stages. In addition to genes, environment, nutrition, and lifestyles, some other causes also include the events of life and our ability to manage them better. Therefore, among the individual factors that determine the response to carcinogens (individual susceptibility), stress should also be counted.

There are some roads in which stress response can follow in promoting carcinogenesis and neoplastic progression. An increase in the production of neurotransmitters and stress hormones, on one hand it can cause an increase of signaling of cell proliferation, mediated by the increase of the growth factors induced in particular by norepinephrine and adrenaline and, on the other hand, with the increase in cortisol, that can cause a dysregulation of the immune response with increased TH2 and TH17 activities which are unsuitable for destroying malignant cells.

On the contrary, the imbalance of the immune response towards TH2-TH17 causes ineffective inflammation leading to the development of metastases that, as it is known, are the cause of death.

5.2.2.5 The state of evidence

The subject on clinical evidence on the relationship between stress and cancer should be analyzed according to two main aspects: the relationship between stress and the start of cancer, and that between post-diagnosis stress and mortality from cancer. There is strong evidence on the relationship between stress and the onset of cancer on animals, that shows an involvement of the immune system in controlling the onset, the growth, and the metastasis of the tumor, in particular of cell-mediated immunity and NK that make up the so-called Th1 circuit, the only one capable of an effective anticancer response.

As far as human research is concerned, the evidence was weak until recently and related to events such as losses and divorces. A recent meta-analysis of the psychobiology group at the University of London, carried out on 167 controlled studies, albeit with all the necessary precautions, concludes that psychosocial stress is related to an increased incidence of cancer, a worse prognosis, and an increase in mortality. In particular, depression seems to be a key factor in opening doors to disease.

Stronger evidence emerges in the post-diagnosis phase. A recent review of the studies concluded that psychological distress in the peri- and post-diagnostic phase depresses cell-mediated immunity (Th1), which instead is supported by measures of psychological and social support. Of particular note are two recent works: one of the University of Hamburg and the other of the University of Ohio.

The German study assessed the effects of psychosocial support on a group of patients with cancer compared to the control group. Ten years later, between the two groups resulted in a statistically significant difference in survival: 21.3% in the treatment group versus 9.6% in the control group. The difference also persists by removing the subjects that resulted from the calculation not to suffer from cancer or suffering from a benign form.

The American study followed 229 women operated for breast cancer which, before starting chemotherapy, radiotherapy, and other planned therapies, were randomly divided into two groups: one for medical supervision and the other as well for medical control but with the addition of participation in a stress management program, carried out in small groups (8-12 people per group) and conducted by two psychologists.

The program included a one and a half-hour of weekly session for the first four months and then a monthly session for the next eight months (in total 26 sessions for 39 working hours). In each session, deep relaxation techniques were practiced, and problem-solving strategies were discussed, both about psychological or physical nature (pain, fatigue). Operators have greatly emphasized the change in people's lifestyles, urging insertion of physical activity into everyday life, good nutrition, and the use of anti-stress techniques.

The verification was carried out 13 years after the starting of the disease and the result is that the patients who had attended the stress management program were found to have a lower frequency of relapses and a greater survival than the group subjected only to the classic controls from doctors. This study, carried out very carefully, highlights the following consideration: stress management reduces relapses, and increases survival.

It is important to note that all participants have undergone blood exams, mammography, and medical visits every six months for the first five years and then every year. This allowed scholars to monitor the evolution of each individual step by step and verify, for example, that several months before the appearance of recurrence, it was possible to notice an alteration in the inflammatory sense of the immune system. The structure of the immune system, in fact, is the key factor in the evolution of tumor disease.

Another particularly important study, conducted by the University of Chicago, was built on 80 operated women who had been diagnosed with breast cancer, highlights that stress management changes the structure of the immune system. The sample was divided into two groups: one followed an eight weeks course, with a weekly session of two and a half hours each of learning anti-stress and meditative techniques; the other instead acted as a control.

After surgery and before starting the experiment, all patients have been studied with various tools to evaluate the quality of life, the level of stress (through the analysis of cortisol, the main stress hormone), and the level of their immune system (by measuring some cytokines and the activity of some cells).

At this stage, all participants had a low score on the quality of life, high levels of stress, and an overall depressed immune system. By the middle of the meditation course, some important changes were already visible, which then consolidated at the end of the course and in the subsequent check after 3 months. How meditation improves the immune system in patients with cancer? The women who had learned to meditate had a higher relative score to quality of life, with cortisol levels significantly lower than others.

This study showed in "meditators" a very quick ability to recover an immune profile from a healthy person, or rather of a person who is able to hold off, through the Th1 immune circuit, the spontaneous formation of neoplastic cells. When this protective immunity is active, in the blood there are high levels of some molecules (interferon-gamma) and low of others (IL-10 and IL-4). Well, the women who participated in the meditation group had exactly this profile, unlike the others that instead had those values upside down.

5.2.2.6 Stress and immune dysregulation pathologies: the example of the skin

The skin has its own stress system, which operates both independently and in connection with the central stress system. Physical factors related to environment and emotional stress activate the central system, which can alter skin physiology through the cutaneous stress system, which, in turn, can feed back, influencing the central system.

The skin (keratinocytes and melanocytes) has all the enzymatic "machinery" to produce stress hormones: ACTH and -MSH (-Melanocyte-Stimulating Hormone) from POMC (Pro-opiomelanocortin), cortisol from cholesterol. It is relevant to observe that both MSH and cortisol, in addition to having a powerful anti-inflammatory action, also act in the alteration of the barrier and in dysregulation of the immune response.

In the skin we find all the cells of both natural and acquired immunity. They are residential cells: mastoids, Langherans cells, dendritic cells of the dermis, macrophages, T lymphocytes, NK cells. They are circulating cells: basophils, eosinophils, neutrophils, T, and B lymphocytes. But also, epithelial cells such as keratinocytes and melanocytes are an active part of the immune response as they release antimicrobial peptides and inflammatory interleukins.

In short, the skin is an extensive and integrated psycho-neuro-endocrine-immune network. On this basis, it is possible to finally explain the ancient and innumerable observations that link mental distress to the onset and aggravation of skin pathologies on an inflammatory basis.

The skin-brain connection and the mutual influence of the psyche-brain and the skin systems find convincing explanations in the so-called "neurogenic inflammation mediated by stress." The peripheral nerve fibers, in fact, both of the adrenergic and noradrenergic and sensory types, release peptides that can modulate in an inflammatory sense the activity of the cutaneous immune system.

In the animal model, it is widely documented that a psychological stress causes the activation of cutaneous inflammation mediated by peripheral nerve fibers through an increase in CRH peptides (a hormone that releases corticotrophin, master signal of the stress axis activation) and NGF (Nervous Growth Factor) that cause an activation of mast cells (immune cells with high inflammatory power which are also responsible for typical urticaria lesions).

In humans, evidence shows a close link between skin innervation, NGF production, and course of the psoriatic plaque: in the plaque we find a high expression of NGF and an increase in the nerve fibers that make up probably the supply channel of inflammation. In fact, if the damaged area is de-nerved, the skin lesion disappears.

Ultimately, we can conclude that chronic psychic stress negatively affects the balance of the immune system, exposing the body to numerous and important immune-mediated or immune-related diseases.

Chapter 6 - Pain in fibromyalgia as a biopsychosocial model of chronic pain

6.1 Introduction

In the biomedical field, the definition of a pathology is basically a cultural process, where identification and illustration of the characteristics that define a pathology are the subject of a logical synthesis process, capable of distinguishing that certain clinical picture from other pathologies. This is intended to allow the clinician its identification and to implement therapeutic strategies aimed at its etiopathogenesis.

Unfortunately, although chronic pain has been defined as a chronic invalidating pathology with the dignity of autonomy from pathologies that can have primitively determined its appearance, it escapes this identification process.

Even more elusive is the clinical picture defined by the American College of Rheumatology (ACR) as fibromyalgia and basically characterized by a wide-spread chronic pain and tenderness which, in 75% of cases, is accompanied by symptoms such as fatigue, unrefreshing sleep, morning stiffness, and with paraesthesia, irritable colon, disability, in another 25% of cases.

The frequent overlap of symptoms between fibromyalgia as

defined from ACR and a broad spectrum of systemic syndromes, such as chronic fatigue syndrome and various psychogenetic pathologies, or localized such as myofascial syndrome and irritable colon, have raised huge controversies over the real existence of fibromyalgia as a specific pathology.

For this reason, fibromyalgia has been branded somewhat provocatively as a mental construction: "When a patient has tuberculosis, it means that he has tuberculosis, whether this has been diagnosed or not. The same goes for cancer, rheumatoid arthritis, etc. This does not apply to fibromyalgia. Nobody has fibromyalgia until he is diagnosed."

The diagnosis of fibromyalgia is still so inaccurate to push one of the authors of ACR diagnostic criteria for fibromyalgia to publish an editorial in which he critically wonders if 66% of wrong diagnoses do not suggest abandoning the use of these criteria.

In the early 90s, a consensus conference gave birth to a document (The Copenhagen Declaration) which stated that fibromyalgia is part of a wider syndrome including headache, bruxism, irritable bowel, sleep disturbance, dysmenorrhea, depression, anxiety, increased sensitivity to cold, Raynaud's phenomenon, legs without rest, atypical pictures of sensitivity disorders (numbness, paranesthesia, etc.), feeling of weakness, excessive muscle fatigue, cognitive disorders, neuro-vegetative and neuroendocrine alterations.

As you can see, the result was an impressive list of syndromes and symptoms which, if possible, widened even further the spectrum of overlapping between fibromyalgia and other clinical entities, almost throwing back the fibromyalgia in the cauldron of the so-called psychosomatic diseases.

More recently, the OMERACT-8 and OMERACT-9 working groups have tried to establish a distinctive core set for the diagnosis of fibromyalgia, to be applied both in trials and in clinical routine, as well as outcome measures useful for evaluating the real therapeutic efficacy of the various treatments proposed according to the core diagnostic set.

Furthermore, possible objective markers have been defined for diagnosis, with the aim of critically reviewing the data present in the literature on the appearance of cognitive dysfunctions related to fibromyalgia.

Over 70% of the participants in OMERACT-8 agreed that it was essential to evaluate pain in every clinical trial, as well as fatigue, sleep disturbances and that aspects such as cognitive disorders and depression should only be so in certain contexts. Other symptoms, such as stiffness and anxiety as well as neuroimaging and all biological markers, were identified as important research areas, whose data currently available do not allow their use and evaluation in a clinical and instrumental diagnostic core set.

Paradoxically, it is possible to notice how the symptoms that must always be reported are the most clinically evident (pain, fatigue, and sleep), while on the clinical level, what seems most interesting would be the psychological profile and the corresponding functional framework (which instead come more referred to as search items).

OMERACT-9's conclusion was, on one hand, substantially a confirmation of what is attested by OMERACT-8, that is, because of the symptomatic variety, a diagnosis of fibromyalgia can't be achieved without a multidimensional evaluation of the symptoms and, on the other hand, that a correct diagnosis cannot be separated from the functional and psychological profiles impact of these patients.

It is important to note that remarkable steps forward have been made since the first definition of fibromyalgia and that it is available now a greater diagnostic accuracy. However, there is not yet a precise and sure link between semeiological expression - both in terms of symptoms and in terms of their importance - and a clear identification of pathology as defined in chapter opening.

To be provocative, we have now gone from an "undifferentiated" collection to an attempt of a "differentiated" collection of symptoms and signs. Certainly, more ecological, but still far from an acceptable nosological safety.

6.2 The biopsychosocial model of pain

In addition to pain, the absolute ruler of the clinical picture, it is recognized and accepted that fibromyalgia is characterized by two other pivotal symptoms: muscle fatigue and sleep disturbances. A further step in understanding fibromyalgia could therefore be the recognition of a common origin of these symptoms or, more reasonably, the recognition of possible shared pathophysiological mechanisms by the three major fibromyalgia symptoms, as a unifying basis of the pathology.

The idea that is developing in this context is that fibromyalgia is a specific clinical picture of more extensive and complex changes affecting the central nervous system, called sensitization, to define an alteration of the excitation regulation mechanisms (increased) and inhibition (reduced) along the sensor-motor chain.

The basic idea that is evolving is that fibromyalgia can be a specific framework generated by larger and more complex changes in the sensitivity of the central nervous system, where all the components of the sensorimotor chain can be involved in multiple and different levels. In this context, fibromyalgia has been redefined as a "dysfunctional syndrome" (DS) or, more recently, as a "central sensitization syndrome" (CSS). Despite the semantic diversity of the definitions (sensitization vs dysfunction), both allude to a biopsychosocial model of the disease.

Such a model can truly represent a useful paradigm to provide an appropriate terminology for understanding the extreme proteiformity of fibromyalgia symptoms and related conditions. In all of these, sensitization or dysfunction in the central nervous system would allow a homogeneous understanding of nature and symptomatic overlap with a common pathophysiological link, rather than considering them as independent and different conditions, with possible areas of clinical overlap.

Within this context, there is increasing evidence that the everyday factors of stress play a crucial role in the etiology of fibromyalgia, both as risk factors and as aggravation/keeping factors. Subjects with fibromyalgia report more frequently traumatic experiences in childhood, both of healthy subjects and of subjects affected by other pathologies, with a high prevalence of lack of affection (48%) and physical abuse (23%).

Moreover, the cases of sexual abuse (10%) did not appear to differ statistically from those detectable in a comparison sample not affected by fibromyalgia. Although these data can suggest that hostile experiences in childhood play a role as factors of risk in the development of fibromyalgia, the relationship between hostile experiences in childhood and fibromyalgia in adults seems to be more complex. In fact, documented cases of abuse and neglect during childhood do not seem to be predictive elements for the development of painful syndromes. However, it is important to note how painful syndromes clinically unexplainable are often associated with abuses suffered in childhood age.

An etiopathogenetic link between fibromyalgia and stressors is suggested by the evidence that a high occupational stress is linked to a risk of two to four times greater for the development of fibromyalgia, as well as the presence of a high comorbidity between fibromyalgia and the so-called Post-Traumatic Stress Disorder (PTSD). Patients with fibromyalgia show a higher prevalence of PTSD than the general population (6%), and similar to that reported in Vietnam veterans and victims of natural disasters or road accidents.

Strangely, and in apparent conflict with what has been said, it has not been found a significant change in the prevalence of fibromyalgia among the victims of the terrorist attack on the twin towers of the World Trade Center in New York on 11 September 2001. Failure to find an increased incidence of fibromyalgia could have been determined by the enormous pathos and social solidarity that has developed in the American population after the terrorist attack, but it can also point out the fact that stressors must have a strong personal meaning to be perceived as risk factors by individuals. However, it is important to note that 49% of individuals with PTSD fall under the ACR classification for fibromyalgia, differently of 5% of patients with severe depression.

The major symptom of fibromyalgia remains chronic diffuse pain: lasting three months or more, it involves all four limbs as well as the back as a whole. Almost two thirds of patients, if questioned, report warning "Pain everywhere." This description of the pain, felt in every part of the body, was considered of pivotal importance in differentiating fibromyalgia from other conditions.

Pain, despite this ubiquitous presence, is more frequently referred to the points reported by the ACR. Another salient feature of pain in fibromyalgia is its distribution that, from the point of view of innervation, does not meet the criteria of anatomical nervous distribution or regional distribution, not being referred to a specific structure, for example, osteon-articular.

This characteristic often leads the clinician to a hasty somatization diagnosis or worse, of psychogenic pain. Just as frequently, the description of pain leads to describe it as a myalgia, suggesting that its origin is from muscle or periosteum. However, in a sub-group of patients, the reported pain is more pronounced in joint regions, without however any sign of flogistic interest.

Even using pain detection questionnaires such as "McGill Pain Questionnaire," the clinical data of an increased spatial distribution emerge, a greater descriptive richness of pain than all other pathologies, with a number by far greater of pain descriptors than other types of pain.

In patients with fibromyalgia, pain can be described as a combination of adjectives such as: "ardent, burning, tingling, like a shock, a stab, sharp, deep, like a cut, and with the feeling of being bruised everywhere."

From the etiopathogenetic point of view, the semantic characteristics of fibromyalgia would include signs and symptoms such as allodynia, causalgia, hyperalgesia, and skin hyperpathy: characteristics typically referred to chronic neuropathic pain. The characteristics of pain are:

- Allodynia -> Pain caused by a normally painless stimulus;

- Causalgia -> Pain referred to as burning;

- Hyperalgesia -> Excessive sensitivity to pain. It is characterized by slow raising and persistence of sensation;

- Persistent pain -> Persistence of pain after a painful stimulus;

- Spatial summation -> A painless stimulus repeated in space becomes painful;

- Temporal summation -> A long-lasting or repeated painless stimulus it becomes painful;

- Skin hyperpathy -> By dragging a needle over the skin, you feel more on the afflicted dermatomes;

- Tenderness -> Sensitivity to palpation during the physical examination.

Chronic pain, as defined by the International Association for the Study of Pain (IASP), has a very significant psychological component, and it is always accompanied by an emotional dimension (feeling of unpleasantness). This aspect is recognized and underlined in fibromyalgia, where the emotional picture is extremely developed together with negative cognitive aspects such as attentive and memory deficit.

All aspects described, both in the definition of the pain of the IASP and in the fibromyalgia symptoms description provided by the ACR, refer to a biopsychosocial model in which emotion, selective attention, learning phenomena, and memory can induce changes in the central nervous system with some sort of continuous re-modulation of pain sensitivity and perception. This re-modulation can take place in both directions, since pain is also capable of modifying many emotional, behavioral, and cognitive components.

The neurotransmitters involved in this ongoing re-modulation include serotonin, noradrenaline, the endogenous opiates system, gamma-aminobutyric acid, and dopamine. Clinically the concept of central sensitization in fibromyalgia is based on the fact that these conditions (chronic fatigue syndrome, psychogenic syndrome, myofascial pain, irritable bowel syndrome, etc.) May be present in the same group of patients in different combinations of symptoms and severity, in full absence of both micro- and macro tissue damage. However, on the contrary, the same pathologies can share the same central and neuroendocrine nervous alterations.

With indirect confirmation, there is the fact that all these pathologies can respond to a similar group of centrally acting drugs like antidepressants, thus suggesting one or more common central mechanisms. Central sensitization, therefore, can be the common pathogenic junction in a large group of syndromes.

The main syndromes related to the so-called central sensitization system (CSS) are:

- Fibromyalgia

- Chronic Fatigue Syndrome

- Tension-type migraine

- Headache

- Irritable bowel syndrome

- Primary dysmenorrhea

- Myofascial pain syndrome

- Temporomandibular dysfunction

- Restless legs syndrome

- Periodic limb disorder

6.3 Pathophysiological aspects of sensitization of the nervous system

The phenomenon of sensitization, the fibromyalgia, is characterized by hyperalgesia, allodynia, expansion of the receptive field, and by one unpleasant quality of the painful post-stimulus with the persistence of a sensation of burning, throbbing, tingling, numbness. Sensitization is not always linked to central nervous mechanisms as the peripheral nervous system, and the receptor itself may be involved in this process.

Tissue inflammation, also caused by minor trauma, induces in traumatized tissue the production of the so-called "inflammatory soup" of which, among others, some are the bradykinin, the histamine, the cascade of prostaglandins, and the substance P (SP). These pro-algogenic substances activate the transmission along the A-delta fibers and the afferent C-fibers and a contemporary and progressive sensitization of the psychic receptors.

This reduced receptor excitability threshold causes the increase of the afferential barrage on the so-called Wide Dynamic Range neurons (WDR) of the spinal cord on which both nociceptive fibers and not make synapse. In the so bombarded spinal cord, numerous neurotransmitters are activated: substance P, NGF (nerve growth factor), CGRP (calcitonin gene-related peptide), VIP (vasoactive intestinal peptide), glutamate, aspartate, and various centrally derived neurotrophic factors (brain-derived neurotrophic factors).

These events - the sensitization of the receptor, the bombing on WDR, and the production of excitatory neurotransmitters in the spinal cord - are capable of inducing a prohalogen change in post-synaptic cell responses, also inducing the development of sensitization phenomena at central level.

These changes include an increase in the permeability of the membrane with increased intracellular calcium flow, activation of the proteinkinase (PK), and an increased expression of c-fos as well as the activation of NMDA receptors.

Currently, some immunological mechanisms have also been highlighted, as they can intervene both in the transmission of the painful stimulus and in establishing a central sensitization. Activation of glial-type immune cells in the central nervous system can induce a pro-inflammatory cytokine release to facilitate the starting of central sensitization and, clinically, a diffuse muscle pain.

This relationship between sensitization, immune system, and pain has also been shown in reverse: chronic muscle pain can induce immunological modifications, and through these, a central sensitization able to self-maintain muscle pain.

Central sensitization can therefore be greatly influenced by peripheral nociceptive barrage generators (for example, arthritic phenomena) but also by many other factors, both endogenous and exogenous. These other factors include neuro-vegetative reactivity, genetic factors, endocrines factors (e.g., a relative hypo-function of the adrenal and a reduced production of Growth Hormone (GH), inter-current viral infections, obstinate insomnia, as well as particularly stressors environmental stimuli such as noise, light, chemicals, etc.) And psychological stress.

From this point of view, it is important to underline that the various etiopathogenetic factors associated with central sensitization syndromes (including fibromyalgia) must not only be seen as "multifactorial" but also as "multiplying factors" in a bio-psychophysical sense. The various factors in combination can amplify and support central sensitization, as well as cause the presence of certain symptoms through their interactive and synergistic actions.

For example, the genetic predisposition in combination with central sensitization may be indicative of a possible development of temporomandibular dysfunction (TMD) in asymptomatic subjects; a dysfunction of the hypothalamic-pituitary-adrenal axis, in combination with psychological stress, can predict the development of a symptomatology widespread pain; car accident trauma, associated with pre-existing psychological factors can cause the onset of fibromyalgia. Same genetic factors have been documented in fibromyalgia as a condition of central sensitization.

Symptoms often referred to by fibromyalgia patients, not included in the core set for diagnosis of fibromyalgia, but associated with CSS:

1. Symptoms affecting the muscular and skeletal system

    a. Generalized stiffness

    b. Muscle cramps

c. Functional alterations of the temporomandibular joint

d. Fatigue, reported hypotonia, and a feeling of paralysis

2. Walking and balance symptoms

   a. Precarious balance, pseudo-ataxia

   b. Awkward running, tendency to stumble

   c. Difficulty with tandem gait

3. Sensory symptoms

   a. Headache or other forms of migraine

   b. Perceptual distortions (eg: bloated sensation)

   c. Itching (also ocular)

   d. Sensory overload phenomena (eg: photophobia; hyperacusis; cacosmia)

   e. Loss of cognitive map

   f. Feeling of tightness in the chest

4. Symptoms affecting the neuroendocrine and vegetative system

   a. Marked weight variation

   b. Hot/cold intolerance

   c. Excessive sweating

   d. Excessive dryness (ocular, vaginal mucosa, etc.)

5. Cognitive and neuropsychological symptoms

   a. Changes in mood

   b. Reactive depression

   c. Anxiety

   d. Difficulty in recovering speech

   e. Confusion and confabulation

   f. Difficulty in short-term memory

6. Cardiovascular and respiratory symptoms

a. Neuro-mediated hypotension

b. Fainting or dizziness

c. Palpitations and tachycardia

d. Water retention

e. Raynaud's phenomena

f. I see them

g. Dyspnea (hunger for air)

7. Digestive system

a. Feeling of a lump in the throat with difficulty
    in swallowing

b. Nausea

c. Stomach ache

d. Abdominal pain

e. Dyspepsia

8. Urinary system

a. Irritable bladder

b. Stranguria

9. Reproductive system

   a. Dysmenorrhea

   b. Premenstrual syndrome or irregular periods

   c. Loss of libido or impotence

   d. Anorgasmia

6.4 Conclusions

The idea that is evolving of a sensitization or dysfunction of
the central nervous system, based on the multifactorial
interaction of biological, psychological, and social aspects,
it can be a conceptual framework to be taken into
consideration for the diagnostic activity of fibromyalgia and
related syndromes, as it is done in our daily outpatient
practice.

A better understanding of the biopsychosocial model in the
context of fibromyalgia, and more generally, of chronic pain,
is certainly an advancement in understanding the
proteiform symptomatology of fibromyalgia, and it
represents a huge stimulus to guide doctors to a wider
understanding of the pathophysiological changes linked to

that, both as regards to its cardinal symptoms and to the less frequent ones. Such an approach can really help to minimize incorrect diagnoses and to improve the therapeutic setting.

In this context, the biopsychosocial model can be seen as a bridge between a set of generic symptoms (considered by the doctor as annoying because they cannot be framed in a precise context of illness), a more correct taxonomy, and a pharmacological therapy tailored to the actual needs of the patient aimed at minimizing them the side effects.

Chapter 7 - Allergology and stress: from the allergic patient to the panallergic one

7.1 Introduction

The concept of the "patients allergic to everything" was introduced in the 80s, and it really was a pioneering approach as it was based on both the theory of the mental origin of the manifestations of disease and on the approach centered on the individual as a whole.

In the following years, specialists in allergology and immunology started to see the "panallergic" patients parading in their clinics, and we all realized how little scientific attention was given to them and, very often, we behave accordingly, making it a syndrome with anecdotal contents but not really based on any scientific doctrine.

Over the years, we have built a mental identikit of the panallergic patient (middle-aged women with nonspecific disorders attributable to the psycho-psychiatric sphere) that we diverted to other specialists increasing the discomfort of patients and subjecting them to increasingly complex and poorly resolving diagnostic procedures.

Various aspects have changed over the past decade. First of all, the percentage of these patients has sharply increased, as also documented by the literature.

From a review of the personal case history of the last year, the patients can be called panallergic represent 3.7% of the total, approaching the percentage of other pathologies more strictly codified on a scientific level, such as a true allergy to drugs (in personal cases at 4.2%), imposing a change of approach in the management of these patients: from anecdotal to taking care of patients in both diagnostic and therapeutic terms.

The main symptoms of the "panallergic" patient are:

- Malaise, psychomotor agitation, feeling of impending doom;

- Vertigo, asthenia, lethargy, headache;

- Referred urticaria (very often episodic and migrant);

- Itching, widespread or more often localized, in this case to the scalp, to a limb, in the anus-genital region;

- Paresthesia affecting the lips and tongue;

- Sense of glottal obstruction, aphonic;

- Sense of chest tightness, heart pounding, angina-like pain;

- Transient amaurosi (total loss of vision), visual changes (glittering scotomas, etc.);

- Olfactory illusions (mainly hyper osmic), o metallic taste sensation o however anomalous;

- Nausea, abdominal pain, bladder and rectal tenesmus (spasm of the sphincter);

- Limbic-myalgia and motor deficit of the limbs lower.

The main signs of the "panallergic" patient are:

- Tachycardia, elevation of blood pressure arterial, tremors;

- Tachypnea, poly-apnea, "sighing breath." cough;

- Blank sneezing, watery rhinorrhea, especially in the morning;

- Pallor, diaphoresis, rash, hives, asymptomatic dermographism (abnormal skin reactivity);

- Labial and/or eyelid angioedema;

- Incontinence of urine and/or loose stools;

- Transient loss of consciousness.

Examining main symptoms and signs that distinguish such patients, we can find vague and nonspecific symptoms but able to significantly alter the patient's quality of life, above all if these symptoms are daily.

In recent years, the identikit of these patients has also changed radically: male patients have appeared, patients have now a higher cultural background, and different phenotypes can be recognized (allergy at all drugs, all foods, all chemists, etc.), but it is mainly on a formal level that the turning point occurred: the panallergic patient passes casually from the concept of allergy to the concept of intolerance, bringing them together.

While for doctors the concepts of allergy and idiosyncrasy/intolerance have pathophysiological and, therefore, very different diagnoses and therapies, for the patient there are no substantial distinctions between the two definitions, since it is only a formal and secondary aspect.

Substance plays a secondary role, it is the "format" that counts, the presentation, the symptoms, the self-diagnosis from abundant internet browsing, or chat rooms. In this environment the discomfort and therefore the "panallergic" syndrome are formalized by the patient itself, before the medical practice.

We move, in fact, in a historical-cultural context that increasingly adopts expressive simplification methods, perhaps for a kind of lexical self-defense from the complexity. It is on this basis that probably well-established keywords in our common lexicon (allergy) are used in a broader and more comprehensive context: everything that is potentially harmful to our body.

Very often alongside this concept of enlarged allergy, we also find the concept of "immune system weakness": the immune system is weakened by stress, physical activity, work, and easily becomes prey to invisible but very strong attackers.

The two formal concepts, together, synergize in communicational terms, both externally and in the inner world of the patient, and are at the basis of many clinical stories of panallergic patients. The purpose of this chapter is to provide the reader with concrete clinical experiences in which to trace a possible strategic procedure in the diagnostics management of these patients. The work is not intended to provide a detailed examination of pathophysiological research in progress on this topic, as this can already be found in the literature.

Here are presented four clinical cases representing different phenotypes of panallergic patients. Some sensitive data of the clinical cases set out below have been carefully modified to protect patient privacy.

Clinical case 1

Male patient, 23 years old, comes to the observation for suspected drug allergy. In the medical request is indicated as "multiple allergy to drugs." The patient reports a complex story: an episode of aspirin allergy in early childhood, then a history of repeated allergic skin situations after taking antibiotics in the category of beta-lactams (ampicilin and amoxycillin), an episode referable to intake of clarithromycin, other episodes related to taking anti-cough preparations and an episode of "anaphylactic shock" after the first and only dental anesthesia procedure.

The episodes are narrated by the patient with great emotional participation, the abundance of details, but no episode is documented by a medical report by an emergency room admission, not even the episode reporting the anaphylactic shock. The patient also points out that he has a ticklish cough during almost all the year, probably allergic.

This detail is interpreted by us as a request for help from the subject. A precise diagnostic path focused on respiratory allergy is then defined for him, which the patient accepts. In subsequent diagnostic visits, he is told that simple screening tests (skin tests and simple spirometry with salbutamol test) do not document a respiratory allergy, and he is therefore offered the possibility to perform an antibiotic exposure test in a day hospital to be able to use it in case of need.

After a few days, the patient, accompanied by the mother, comes to ask for detailed explanations on the exposure test. On that occasion the mother intervenes, explaining a story very similar to that of the son with similar clinical pictures, with awareness spectrum for the same drugs, and curiously with very strong temporal analogies. Another aspect that unites the two is that reactions never take place at the first dosage but invariably at the second or third dosage of the drug, an occasion in which the "maximum and therapeutic" dosage is reached. The mother also explains that she only worked out for herself and for his son a food diet free of drugs that pollute food (aspirin, antibiotics).

Both agree to undergo the same day hospital test and are told that it will be used even a placebo. The mother appears happy to undergo this test with her son. The two patients react in unison to the second placebo tablet, with a showy facial erythema, some strong cough, and a sense of fainting. Any attempt to carefully explain what happened fails. After a few months, a colleague tells me that he met a son and mother allergic to all drugs (all really all!): their description corresponded to that of the patients described above.

The case documents a true panallergic march in which a suspected allergy episode to a drug, possible, but much more likely a mild adverse event in the course of childhood viral infection, it represents the primum movens to build an allergological history. The story is strictly undocumented (although very rich in details), and also episodes defined as severe (first aid, anaphylactic shock) are not supported by any medical records.

Over time, the patient builds an allergic phenotype focused on drugs but always available to expand to other horizons (respiratory allergy and, above all, food allergy), so it is of crucial important to block the false allergy diagnoses to drugs also for this reason.

The most important negative consequence of the establishment of a panallergy situation to drugs lies in the fact that, when there is a real need, the patient becomes difficult to treat. It should be noted that, in some cases, doctors also do their part, carefully avoiding to deepen the diagnostic topics and increasingly narrowing the range of pharmacological categories available to the patient, who, without obvious reasons, becomes increasingly orphaned of drugs and this heightens his fear of getting sick, further feeding his phobias.

Get in touch with the patient and induce him to carry out a specialist diagnostic process appears complex, but very often, it is easier to divert him on marginal paths perceived by the patient as less dangerous, using subsequent meetings opportunities to better re-evaluate and redefine the dominant problem.

In the case of panallergy to drugs, the idea of accumulation dominates as if the drug, endowed with lethal consequences in itself, needs to accumulate. On one side, therefore, we have a patient who feels vulnerable to the harmful action of the drug because they claim to have a weak immune system, and on the other hand, we have a very powerful substance able to bring about healing (life) or death.

In the clinical case described here, the panallergy pathway appears to be dominated by a phobic framework shared between mother and son, in a sort of sadomasochistic relationship focused on the drug experienced as a powerful destructive weapon of relationship, a "pharmacological" path that unites and feeds, potentially with possibilities of infinite evolution (see for example the food diversion). The continuation of the troubled diagnostic process of this couple of unhappy pharmacologists, unfortunately, seems destined to last.

The presented clinical case also demonstrates the diagnostic importance of placebo, often underestimated by doctors, to expose complex situations. This procedure, beyond the many ethical problems, it could represent a solid basis to release the patient from his phobic state and therefore be able to carry out tests of challenge by drawing up a list, even minimal, of well-tolerated drugs; all this to allow patients to face therapies with serenity, even occasional, but necessary.

Clinical case 2

Female patient, 32 years old, comes to the clinical observation complaining about "allergy for all foods." A detailed clinical history documents a very evolutionary clinical picture more complex and rigorous with temporal evolution from childhood to adulthood:

- Childhood bronchial asthma, diagnosed with dust and cat allergy. The patient uses salbutamolo daily, even several times a day, but at the request to show how the device is used, she proves not to know how to use it;

- General food allergy, and in childhood was mainly referred to milk and eggs;

- Allergy to all drugs, with an only probable diagnosis of ampicillin allergy. The patient does not take many drugs since then, and only undergoes "non-harmful" homeopathic treatments;

- From puberty, the appearance of "food allergy" with self-diagnosis of celiac disease, intolerance to milk, yeasts, refined sugars, and gradually other foods (including French cheese). On allergy/food intolerance, the patient is particularly competent, and she presents exhaustive documentation exclusively from esoteric tests (Dria test, Vega test, Cytotest, exam of the hair, etc.), performed on various occasions, all with conflicting diagnoses, but from which the patient extrapolated a copied diet, according to her, from that of a famous American designer who is using only exotic and very expensive ingredients.

The patient runs a beauty center with an adjoining diet center. In fact, she presented herself to the medical observation on the insistence of the mother, who accompanies her demonstrating a lot of concern due to deep asthenia, weight loss of about 10 kg in the last six months, and because she suspects she has an extreme weakness of the immune system.

On physical examination, only a picture of mild rhinitis with hypertrophy of the inferior turbinate, breath is sighing, but without asthma, widespread abdominal tenderness on superficial palpation, and moderate pain evoked in correspondence of the descending colon.

As in the previous clinical case, there is a substantial self-reference, the total absence of documentation, both general and specific aspects. The patient performed an immune-allergic screening in childhood about twenty-five years earlier and gradually added allergies to the initial diagnosis. It does not appear available to follow a diagnostic path, declaring skepticism in the official medicine.

At the end of the visit we ask the patient if she has ever considered the possibility of being also "nickel allergic." Stunned, she can't answer, she stammers: "Maybe... but is it also present in food, right?" and on this curiosity/need to expand her knowledge, she agrees to submit to diagnostic tests for nickel.

The patient is not allergic to nickel, but in the 76 hours necessary to read the patch test she comes subjected to respiratory allergy diagnostics, being non-allergic to pollen or cat nor to dust mites and presenting a very normal spirometry picture. The patient, reassured, decides to abandon salbutamol as needed, but significantly refuses diagnostics for food.

On the basis of this refusal, a series of in vitro investigations are drawn up which are expanded to a small internal check-up, at the insistence of the mother, who repeatedly emphasizes the slimming of her daughter.

Blood chemistry tests do not document lactase deficiency, risk of celiac disease, food allergy, or beta-lactam drugs. Instead, there is a picture of mild iron deficiency anemia and especially the presence of occult blood in the stool.

The patient is quickly subjected to a colonoscopy, which diagnoses Crohn's disease, and is sent to a Gastroenterological Center for the appropriate treatment. In subsequent meetings, the mother reports of various hospitalizations for anorexia in puberty. This case documents how very often food-intolerance can be misleading and, above all, conceal, even for years, important diagnoses.

As in the previous case, the patient lies and builds up a history of allergy/intolerance as a loophole for relevant problems in one's emotional sphere: asthma instead of anxiety, enlarged eating disorders to hide the eating behavior. In the specific case, then, the patient even built a working identity on his own problems and on the skills acquired.

It should be emphasized that the proliferation of diagnostic tests for food intolerances corresponds to an unscrupulous marketing strategy, most managed by non-medical personnel (nutritionists, dieticians, personal trainers, acupuncturists, homeopaths, etc.), and supported by the (para) medical press as well as by pharmacies, nutritionist studies probably heavily funded by the "special food" industry and everyone that has strong and concrete interests in this area.

This healthcare marketing strategy has dramatically increased a "dietary demand" that was already present in our social fabric in the form of collective unease resulting from a distorted cult of the body.

It is true that the patient hardly wants to undergo diagnostic protocols as they are very often invasive, long, and expensive to document their ailments, and they have to take drug therapies, often chronic, with results that are not always positive.

Much easier is to obtain a list of non-tolerated foods: this approach recalls the long and detailed lists of impure animals reported in various passages in the Bible with the consequent indisputable prohibitions and anathemas for those who do not respect them.

By resorting to this strategy, a complex problem is simplified at best. After all, dietary practices belong to many religious cultures (Ramadan for Muslims, the Lent for Christians), and they are an act of purification. The truth is that patients, after an attempt at simplification, realize the uselessness of this approach and resort to medical expertise when they are aware that a more relevant problem underlies everything.

In our personal experience, the common trait to these patients is the abnormal reaction to the stress that is structured over the years towards pictures of chronic masked anxiety.

The outside world represents the real enemy: the outside

world is equipped with deadly weapons (drugs, toxic foods, industrial contaminants, pesticides, antibiotics, atmospheric pollution, the hole in the ozone, etc.) Ready to penetrate inside the body and wreak havoc. In the gloomy world of the gastrointestinal tract, such substances can operate their destruction in an undisturbed way or rather rise and grow. It could be explained in these terms the particular attention paid to certain foods such as milk or yeast, which evoke sexuality, pregnancy, breastfeeding.

In addition to contaminating, drugs and food also get dirty because they are expelled with the feces. It is no coincidence that many of these patients show an obsessive body care that very often takes the form of obsessive-compulsive hygiene practices or declare yearnings of cosmic purity, which very often represent the counterpart to escape from a situation of inner danger.

What better than purify yourself through a diet, simple rigorous, and also fashionable, which eliminates the source of contagion and shift attention from inside to outside.

Clinical case 3

Female patient, 42 years old, comes to the observation for panallergy. The patient reports in great detail that she has problems with air pollution, perfumes, and substances by contact and with all drugs.

The reported symptomatology is tachycardia, a sense of constriction in the throat, difficulty in breathing, erythema itchy hands and feet, increased salivation, feeling faint. The contact and the symptoms are daily, and there is a severe alteration of the patient's quality of life.

She reports that she has performed numerous tests but with discordant and inconclusive results. In one case, hypersensitivity was diagnosed by multiple chemists, but only on clinical findings, and then doctors have proposed to the patient an antidepressant therapy, which she promptly refused.

Among the substances to which the patient claims to be "allergic" is nickel, which is everywhere (air, water, food, detergents, perfumes ...), to which the patient attributes many of her symptoms. We decide to focus on that aspect.

The diagnostics document a mild sensitization for nickel, of doubtful significance, but we decide to continue our path together with the patient. Therefore, some inhalation therapy and a nickel vaccine are prescribed, both with the aim of verifying the possible response to a therapeutic plan built on placebo. In the following month, the patient seems to improve, then a rapid worsening follows, attributed to the nickel vaccine, which is promptly suspended.

In the following months, we see a significant change: the patient gradually shrinks her field of malaise at the workplace only. After six months, in a visit also conducted with a fellow psychologist, she says, dramatically, that she started to suffer from this syndrome after a violence in the workplace. The patient is currently in therapy at a center specializing in posttraumatic disorders, but its symptomatology, although improved in terms of severity, continues.

The case documents how the onset of panallergic cadres, even a severe one, can be connected to significant trauma and the subsequent structuring of a syndrome post-traumatic. In most cases, the patient carefully hides the possible existence of such events, and it seems difficult to find out if not collaborating with a specialist colleague.

It is still not clear what the pathophysiological link is between the psychological situation and the clinical pictures of the patients. Very often, the allergological sensitizations found have even a little diagnostic value, and there is no solid scientific proof that in this group of patients, there is a real basic immune-allergological disorder or a frequency of sensitization higher than that found in the general population.

On the medical level, however, it should be remembered that the immuno-allergological evaluation represents an entrance door for the patient who needs help to clarify its difficulties and that we cannot deny, even if it takes months to be able to build a relationship of trust and the subsequent explanation of the trauma: in these cases, it is possible to theorize the use of a therapeutic trial with the placebo which allows to open the doors of the patient and the clinical case.

Clinical case 4

Male patient, 60 years old, comes to the observation with a request from the dentist to perform skin tests for a suspected allergy to local anesthetics. The colleague has drawn up a short memorandum asking us to take charge of the patient who has been refused by other facilities because panallergic, but urgently needs prosthetic intervention. We reassure the patient that we will consider his case urgently and take prompt action to schedule the day hospital.

To the question "But what are you allergic to?" the patient extracts a package of documentation from a bag of about 200 pages, where tests, visits, hospitalizations in the emergency room were carefully cataloged. All the documentation is photocopied, strictly in chronological order, and some parts are also highlighted in yellow for easy reading. Faced with such unexpected documentation, we took some time to study it carefully. We found that the following diagnoses were given to the patient:

- Hypersensitivity syndrome for multiple chemists;

- Fibromyalgia;

- Chronic fatigue syndrome;

- Allergy to NSAIDs (aspirin);

- Amalgam syndrome;

- Allergy to milk and yeast;

- Hypogonadism;

- Hypothyroidism;

- Chronic EBV infection;

- Intolerance for multiple food additives.

All diagnoses seem to be supported by very sophisticated, diagnostic tests and investigations, but none seems conclusive; on the contrary, there is a total diagnostic dissonance in the various temporal phases of the documentation.

We decide not to take into account the documentation but to focus on the patient by making a clean slate of previous diagnoses. We call him and agree on the diagnostic process only on local anesthetics, extending the time of diagnostics to have the opportunity to visit him with care. On physical examination, the patient is obviously overweight, medium-sized hypertensive, with moderate hepatomegaly, atrophic rhinitis as a result of abuse of vasoconstrictors.

We offer him the local anesthetic exposure test, which was negative (with signs of great relief from the patient), a series of investigations of international interest to better define his immunological and general situation: the patient accepts and emphasizes that "He has a very weak immune system." In the meantime, he was given a restrictive qualitative diet for food additives, a "powerful" antihistamine never used before to protect it from sudden allergic attacks, a premedication for dental care, and availability via e-mail.

The extended evaluation shows the total absence of specific allergic sensitization, the absence of endocrinological, immunological or infectious changes, but a picture of liver steatosis with associated metabolic syndrome with moderate severity: we make a new appointment, but after an adequate interval, to discuss exams and undertaken placebo-therapy. By telephone, the patient says he is very satisfied with the therapy and that he feels much better.

In the next visit, also conducted in this case in collaboration with the psychologist, the truth emerges: after two almost contemporary traumatic events, a mourning and a stormy divorce, the patient has become an ethicist. We also have a suspicion that abuse of illicit substances, but he denies. He is sent for therapy to a specialized center for alcoholism, but we have no longer received his news.

After months, we had the curiosity to re-read the documentation provided by this patient: a treatment with antabuse carried out in a hospitalization had completely escaped years ago, and that hadn't been underlined in yellow!

This case demonstrates how, sometimes, the stories of these patients underlie events of dramatic lives (bereavements, difficult divorces, betrayals, mobbing, stalking, abortions, anaphylactic shocks of family members, car accidents, robberies, tumor diseases to relatives or friends, rape and violence in the family, pedophilia) which play a key role in the construction of a panallergy routes.

The temporal relationship is rarely, like in this case, linear, but much more often, there is a temporal dissociation, which makes the search for the causal link very problematic. The difficulty of the patient to express such difficult and complex situations does the rest. The case also demonstrates how patients provide us with ancillary signals that we understand in almost all cases because we are busy tracing our diagnostic protocols, chasing the box where we want the patient to be inserted.

This case demonstrates, once again, how fundamental multi-specialist collaboration is to define the correct diagnosis and how bad current university teaching is on these topics. It remains difficult to understand why the patient diverted attention to immuno-allergy ailments.

This is likely to be attributed to ease of collect information, to the substantial impossibility of providing certain diagnostic protocols in poorly defined syndromes, but also to the wandering of such patients in centers and structures always ready to provide "alternative" diagnoses.

7.2 Conclusions

Panallergic syndromes are increasing in clinical practice, but we don't know whether this increase is real or only determined by greater diagnostic attention. It is also likely that by moving into an increasingly context marked by social discomfort, by solitude, and strenuous competition, the patient is much more inclined to divert and structure his suffering/stress by focusing on immune-allergological disorders in which his room for maneuver appears likely to be large for the lack of validated diagnostic protocols.

The role of the widely circulated press has not to be underestimated, as it provides such patients with simple self-diagnosis on allergy-intolerance. Intercepting the demand for these "fake allergies" is certainly a challenge for the future, even if it appears difficult in an increasingly marked medical context, where evaluation time and economic aspects are increasingly stringent.

Here are some examples of clinical-operative suggestions that may have a value for the definition of cases of panallergic patients:

- Center the anamnesis not on the symptoms but on the patient;

- Always reassure the patient about his state of health or about "organic" diseases that have escaped from previous investigations;

- Confirm the work of other colleagues or previous diagnoses, focusing on aspects apparently residual but on which the patient is receptive;

- Investigate, with discretion but in depth, on possible traumatic events or conditions of discomfort (never use the word "stress") in its usual life context (work, family, etc.);

- Convince the patient to make a diagnosis of disease by actively involving him in this research, also defining a plausible time span (months);

- Use all the meeting opportunities in the field of diagnostics to search for signals, apparently accessories that the patient throws;

- Use placebo treatments for diagnosis;

- Always emphasize the benefits of not being allergic or intolerant;

- Never use a psychiatric diagnosis;

- In case of diagnosis, provide practical solutions, previously prepared.

However, it seems crucial to work in a team to catch accessory signals and succeed to "open the patient" by building a solid doctor-patient relationship for his involvement in the diagnostic process. Knowledge and application of techniques to manage the doctor-patient relationship currently appear a lot of deficiencies, while it would be desirable to be an integral part of the teaching of the degree course in Medicine.

In our view, both in the diagnostic and in the therapeutic phases, the use of placebo is considered relevant because, beyond ethical considerations, it is an easy tool to be applied, and it is capable of opening unexpected paths.

The relationship between these syndromes and the immune system still remains unsolved. A probable role of genetics has recently been hypothesized, and probably in the future, we will have more concrete answers, making these pathologies less orphaned both on the diagnostic and therapeutic levels.

Chapter 8 - Stress and cardiovascular diseases

8.1 Introduction

Since ancient times people have had the intuition of a link between emotional stress and heart, and long before doctors became interested in this relationship, popular wisdom in many different societies and cultures conveyed the idea that strong emotions could cause sudden death. Common language is also full of expressions such as "he died of a broken heart," "my heart bursts," etc., which allude to this relationship.

In the scientific literature, it is known that acute physical stressors (e.g., surgery interventions, trauma, and intense physical exertion) are triggers of cardiovascular events, and emotional stressors are increasingly recognized as precipitants of such events. It is also known that stressful events influence the pathogenesis of a physical illness, causing negative affective states, for example, feelings of anxiety and depression, which can exert direct effects on biological processes or on behavioral patterns that, in turn, influence disease risk.

Exposure to chronic stress is considered the most harmful risk factor, because it could produce long-term and/or permanent changes in physiological, emotional, and behavioral responses, influencing susceptibility to develop the disease. This includes stressful situations that persist for an extended period (for example, assistance to family members with dementia or degenerative diseases) or traumatic episodes (for example, being a victim of sexual violence).

The existential stressful events that have been most studied in their relations with the onset of cardiovascular disease are the events of loss. The risk of cardiovascular disease also increases among healthy subjects who have experienced traumatic events, such as the death of a child, or who have been exposed to emotional, sexual, physical abuse during the first years of life. In a similar mode, recurrent cardiovascular events and mortality increase with a perceived stressed life, work overload, marital stress, and social isolation among people with pre-existing cardiovascular diseases.

The meta-analysis highlights that the risk associated with psychological factors is similar in magnitude to that of other important and well known clinical risk indicators. This chapter attempts to illustrate the state of the art on the relationship between stress and cardiovascular disease, widely documented to date, although the term stress has been used over the years and by several researchers with different meanings, and this makes it difficult to reach definitive conclusions.

8.2 Stress and psychosocial factors

A worldwide demonstration of the interaction between stress and heart attack is provided by the INTERHEART study. The study was born from the observation that although over 80% of the global cardiovascular diseases fall on poorer countries, knowledge of risk factors comes largely from most developed countries. The effect of the same risk factors on coronary heart disease in many areas of the world remains unclear, despite international studies being conducted.

The INTERHEART study investigated the relationship between psychosocial factors and the risk of myocardial infarction in 25,000 people from 50 countries, using a case-control design with 11,000 patients with a first myocardial infarction and 13,500 controls matched by gender and age, in 260 centers in Asia, Europe, Middle East, Africa, Australia, North and South America.

Psychosocial stress was investigated through simple questions regarding perceived stress at work, at home, financial stress, and life events over the past year. More questions have investigated the *locus of control* and the presence of depression. The locus of control indicates how an individual believes the events of his life are produced by his behavior or actions, or by external causes independently from his will.

There are two types: High (or Internal: individuals who believe in their own ability to control events), and Low (or External: individuals who believe that life events are not the result of the direct exercise of personal ability, but rather due to unpredictable external factors such as the luck or fate). The results indicate that people with myocardial infarction reported a higher prevalence of all four stressors and depression symptoms; in addition, a high locus of control has emerged as a protective factor.

The proliferation of systematic studies and reviews has been observed over the past ten years, reported by guidelines and books on cardiovascular disease, which show scientific evidence of a close etiological and prognostic link between psychological variables and cardiovascular diseases.

Numerous studies have shown that some factors, called psychosocial factors, considerably influence the coronary heart disease, in the sense that these factors are associated with a higher probability that atherosclerosis or an unfavorable cardiac event occurs. In particular, the latest European guidelines on cardiovascular disease prevention show that the low socio-economic level, social isolation and the lack of social support, work and family stress, negative emotions, including depression and hostility, are the psychosocial factors that have been shown to influence the risk of developing ischemic heart disease and to worsen the clinical course and prognosis of patients with ischemic heart disease.

Here is the list of the psychosocial risk factors supported by scientific evidences reported in literature that will be further discussed in the following paragraphs:

- Low socio-economic level;

- Social isolation and lack of social support;

- Work and family stress;

- Depression;

- Anxiety;

- Hostility and anger;

- Type D personality (Distressed).

8.2.1 Psychosocial risk factors

8.2.1.1 Low socio-economic level

Numerous large studies have shown that men and women with low socio-economic level (defined as low education, low income, having a low-level job, or living in a poor residential area) have a high risk of mortality, both general and coronary.

8.2.1.2 Social isolation and lack of social support

Some studies have focused attention on the qualitative aspect of social support, evaluating the so-called social network. Numerous data allow today to quantify the risk of ischemic heart disease in socially isolated individuals, as increased, on average, 2-3 times. A supportive social network would constitute, instead, a cardio-protective factor, as scholars have stressed the role of social isolation, self-accusation, avoidance, and painful life events, identifying high-stress levels in 75% of heart attacks.

People who are isolated or unrelated to others increase the risk of premature death from coronary heart disease. Likewise, the lack of social support leads to a decrease in survival and to a worsening of the prognosis in subjects with clinical manifestations already in place. Social support can be an important protective factor in dealing with chronic stress and disease.

8.2.1.3 Work and family stress

The idea that a psycho-social negative workplace is a factor of risk for coronary heart disease is generally well accepted, but a precise definition of the "toxic" components is not yet available.

Over the past two decades, two theoretical models of chronic work psychosocial stress have received attention in international research: the model "demand-control" or "job strain" focused on control, and the "effort-reward imbalance" focused on reward, that is, on the employment contract. The first model postulates that a combination of job characteristics (high demands in combination with low job control, in which the individual cannot moderate the pressure caused by high demands) elicits recurring responses of stress. In the second model, the conflict between high and low workload reward (in terms of money, esteem, aspects related to promotions, low working security) produces a condition of distress. These two models integrate with each other.

Recent reviews indicate that in most cases, both models and their individual components are associated significantly with a high relative risk of fatal or non-fatal cardiac events. In particular, a meta-analysis estimated an approximately 50% increase in cardiovascular risk associated with high levels of work stress.

A systematic review indicates that high psychological demands, lack of social support, experiment tensions without support are risk factors for ischemic heart disease among men, however, the studies involving women are too few to draw conclusions. A recent study indicates that overtime is associated with coronary heart disease risk regardless of conventional risk factors.

As for family stress, some studies show that conflicts, crises, and long-term stressful family living conditions increase the risk of coronary heart disease, especially in women.

8.2.1.4 Depression

Numerous systematic reviews and meta-analyses have shown that clinical depression and depressive symptoms predict coronary heart disease and worsen coronary heart disease prognosis. Stressful life events have been associated with depressive disorder as well as depressive symptoms, and about 25% of people who have had stressful events develop depression. The perceived social support seems to counteract the negative effects of depression, while the lack of support reinforces its adverse effects.

8.2.1.5 Anxiety

Two recent meta-analyses show that anxiety is an independent risk factor for coronary heart disease and subsequent events after a heart attack. Recent epidemiological studies indicate that panic attacks increase the risk of cardiovascular events.

8.2.1.6 Hostility and anger

Hostility is a multidimensional construct, which includes cognitive, affective, and behavioral components, characterized by negative thoughts and attitudes towards the others, difficult to define, and it is now considered the type A "toxic" component. The concept of type A personality was introduced in the 60s, observing common behavior characteristics in many patients with coronary artery disease. People with Type A behavior are characterized by ambition, competitiveness, anger, and hostility.

Large-scale prospective studies conducted in the 70s and 80s on healthy subjects showed that type A individuals presented a significantly increased risk to develop coronary artery disease or heart attack, but subsequently, a fair number of studies have not confirmed this association. These contradictory results induced to seek a certain component of type A behavior that could be associated with coronary heart disease: this work suggested that anger and/or repressed anger are the pathogenetic components of type A personality.

A recent meta-analysis confirmed that anger and hostility are associated with an increased risk of cardiovascular events in both the healthy population and in the coronary artery patients. However, this effect is less than that observed for depression and anxiety.

8.2.1.7 Type D personalities

Type D personality has been identified as a determining element of psychological distress and as an independent predictor of mortality and morbidity in patients with chronic coronary artery disease, regardless of traditional cardiovascular risk factors. Type D personality is a combination of two dimensions, assumed to be relatively independent of each other: negative affectivity (NA) and social inhibition (SI).

The first refers to the trend to experience negative emotions over time and in different situations; the second is the trend to inhibit emotions and behaviors in social interactions. The author of the construct started from the assumption that it is not experiencing negative emotions in itself, but rather the chronic psychological distress, which results from the negative emotions experienced, to influence physical health.

The first study, which highlighted deleterious effects of the type D personological configuration on health in patients with coronary heart disease, identifies in the type D personality an independent predictor of cardiac events. The enlargement of the sample and the extension of follow-up have highlighted, in an important subsequent work, higher mortality in type D versus non-D patients.

Another study confirmed the influence of type D personality

on the clinical course in a selected sample of patients with negative prognosis (left ventricular ejection fraction <50). These studies show that Type D personality is an important long term mortality predictor in patients with coronary artery disease, regardless of biomedical risk factors, and cardiac events in post-infarction patients with negative prognosis.

Some studies show that Type D personality predicts a bad prognosis in patients with coronary artery disease, even after adjustment for depressive symptoms, stress, and anger. A recent Italian study investigated health status, quality of life, coping strategies for patients in cardiology rehabilitation, and the influence of type D personality on the outcome after the discharge from rehabilitation.

It turned out that the D-type personality seems to significantly play a clinically relevant role in the outcome related to psychological health. Patients with type D personalities, compared to subjects with non-D-type personalities, show a significantly higher level of psychological impairment, in terms of anxiety symptoms, depressed mood, perceived psychophysical stress, reduced psychophysical well-being, interpersonal difficulties, social anxiety, and a significantly lower level of satisfaction with the quality of life before and after rehabilitation. Type D personality also appears to be associated with more maladaptive coping strategies.

8.2.2 Stress, psychosocial factors and cardiovascular disease

Psychosocial risk factors do not occur individually, but tend to come together in the same category of subjects or groups, for example, subjects with low socio-economic conditions. In addition to unhealthy lifestyles, such as a smoking habit and inappropriate nutrition, individuals with psychosocial risk factors such as depression most frequently have physiological features involved in the determinism of cardiovascular disease, for example, alterations of the autonomous and endocrine system and indicators of inflammation.

A recent review on the topic shows that psychosocial risk factors act on the sympathetic nervous system and on the hypothalamic-pituitary adrenaline axis, resulting in activation. Such activation can have several effects at the peripheral level that lead to an increase in the state of psychological reactivity of the individual to acute stress, which may add to the effects of chronic stressors, leading to a deterioration in the subject's health.

At a peripheral level, some malfunctions can occur at the autonomous nervous system, insulin-resistance, central obesity, hypertension, inflammation, platelet activation, endothelial function changes, ovarian dysfunctions, decrease in bone density, and somatic effects.

Atherosclerosis is now considered to be the result of a prolonged inflammatory process over time on the walls of the arteries, and this same inflammatory process can be determined by stress. Stress itself is often the cause-effect of other psychosocial risk factors, and it acts on the sympathetic nervous system, on the hypothalamic-pituitary axis, and on the renin-angiotensin system, causing the release of some hormones that are able to lead to an increase in cardiovascular activity, injuries to the endothelium, and which facilitate the adhesion of several types of molecules in the vascular walls (corticosteroids, growth hormone, catecholamine, homocysteine , etc.).

Furthermore, stress is capable of causing lipid oxidation and, if chronic, a hyper-coagulation condition that can easily lead to the production of a thrombus. Finally, there are also other types of responses related to stresses that promote the inflammatory process: activation of macrophages, cytokines production, and other inflammatory mediators, acute phase proteins, etc.

8.3 Role of emotional factors in the beginning of cardiac events

Most research, focused on long-term etiology, has therefore shown that exposure to psychosocial risk factors accelerates the process of atherosclerosis, and the incidence of coronary events increases. There is, however, another way in which emotional triggers could contribute to the beginning of the cardiovascular disease, that is, as a trigger of acute heart disease, such as myocardial infarction, unstable angina, or sudden cardiac death sudden.

Cardiac events typically occur in people with coronary atherosclerosis, and the emotional factors involved in the acute phase are not necessarily the same involved in the long term, as they act on a shorter time span.

A trigger is a stimulus or activity that produces highs physiological or pathophysiological changes that trigger a cardiac event and generally occur in the hours immediately preceding the event. Triggers can take many forms, including physical exertion, heat and cold stress, infections, the use of substances like cocaine.

As for emotions, studies teach us that it is difficult to study emotional triggers of cardiac events with prospective studies, since the occurrence of acute myocardial infarction or sudden cardiac death cannot be expected in advance. So the studies on the emotional trigger of cardiac events are typically retrospective, and two strategies are possible, taking into account both these methods have strengths and limitations:

1. <u>Population-based studies</u>: allow to study the impact

of emotionally stressful events such as natural disasters, terrorist attacks, industrial catastrophes, and sporting events on hospitalizations for acute coronary syndrome or on the occurrence of sudden cardiac death;

2. <u>Studies based on emotions in individuals</u>: they allow you to study individuals after suffering a cardiac event, investigating their stressful experiences in the period preceding the beginning of symptoms. This allows to collect accurate information about emotions.

8.3.1 Population-based studies

Earthquakes are devastating and very stressful experiences, and their effects on acute heart events have been studied in several countries, although they are sometimes observed mixed results. In the 90s, Los Angeles experienced a very strong heartquake, and millions of people were suddenly awakened in the middle of the night.

In the following hours, a number of deaths due to cardiac causes occurred about 6 times higher than in the period immediately preceding the event. Almost one year later, in January 1995, a very intense earthquake struck Japan in the region of Awaji-Hokudan, and in this case, the number of cardiac deaths tripled in the weeks following the earthquake.

It is also a common belief that during the wars, there may be an incidence of deaths from cardiac causes among the civilian population, even if the cause of the number of deaths caused by weapons has been unknown.

In January 1991, during the first Gulf War, the civilian population of Israel was put on alert and equipped with anti-gas masks to defend against attacks with unconventional weapons by Iraqi military forces. The first day of the missile attack, the number of cardiac deaths in Israel increased suddenly and remained elevated throughout the week of the attacks.

An increase in the incidence of acute myocardial infarction and sudden death during the early stages of the Gulf War in 1991 and this was confirmed by a national study in Israel, which, on the day the first missile hit the population, showed a 58% increase in mortality in large part attributable to acute myocardial infarction and sudden cardiac death.

Some studies have also been conducted on the incidence of cardiovascular events after the terrorist attack on the World Trade Center in New York on 11 September 2001; some authors report a statistically significant increase in myocardial infarction, but not of tacky-arrhythmias in the 60 days after the fact; others report that the impact of the event also manifested itself in non-New York patients with defibrillator, not present at the time of the terrorist act, in which, in the 30 days later, the treatment of ventricular arrhythmias increased by 68% compared to the previous 30 days, with a 2.8-fold increase in risk.

Similar results were obtained in a study on New York patients with the same characteristics, leading the authors to conclude that subacute stress may have contributed to promoting arrhythmogenesis.

Finally, big sporting events can be very stressful for fans by acting as a trigger for cardiac events. For example, following an important game of the European football championship of 1996 between France and the Netherlands, which took place ended with a penalty kick, cardiovascular mortality was analyzed in the Dutch population aged 45 or over: a relative risk of death from acute myocardial infarction or higher stroke on the match day for men, while no effect was found on women.

The Authors point out that the effect of the addiction of physical exertion must also be taken into account in these situations, as well as emotional stress and alcohol consumption.

8.3.2 Studies based on emotions in individuals

The first large-scale project for the assessment of emotional triggers in individuals was the Multicenter Investigation of Limitation of Infarct Size (MILIS study) that involved 850 patients interviewed within 18 hours of acute myocardial infarction; the 18% reported emotional upset in the period immediately preceding the onset of symptoms.

In a subsequent study (TRIMM), emotional disturbance, or stress in the hours preceding acute myocardial infarction was reported by 35% of patients. However, other studies have reported much lower levels of emotional triggers, and a more recent meta-analysis of 18 studies concluded that an average 7% of patients report emotional stress immediately preceding the acute event.

However, the interpretation of the studies that merely verify the presence of trigger is burdened by two problems. First, patient stories can be influenced by their attempts to make sense of disease and their beliefs about the causes of heart disease. In fact, stress is often mentioned, both on patients, both from healthy adults, as a major cause of heart disease, and these views can influence memory.

Second, the period of control time has not been tested. If emotional stress occurs frequently in a patient's life, his association with the onset of a syndromecacute coronary artery may be a coincidence. Acute anger is the emotional trigger of acute coronary syndrome that has been studied more widely.

In the Determinants of Myocardial Infarction Onset Study, 2.4% of patients said they were very angry or furious in the 2 hours prior to acute myocardial infarction. A similar result has been reported in the SHEEP study with a clinical cohort of 300 patients: 17.4% reported episodes of acute anger in the 2 hours before the symptoms, associated with conflicts with neighbors, conflicts with family members, and anger during commuting.

Acute work-related stressors were assessed as possible triggers in the SHEEP study. Other studies have assessed emotional stress more generally. For example, emotional disturbances in the two hours preceding the appearance of the cardiac symptoms were reported by a German study, and the increase in myocardial infarction probability after exposure to traffic was indicated by another study.

Acute depression is relevant for both the long-term development of coronary artery disease, both for the prognosis following cardiac events. A recent study has detected the presence of episodes of acute depression and sadness in the 2 hours previous the onset of cardiac symptoms.

In summary, the studies cited provide convergent evidence that they support the role of emotional stimuli in triggering acute coronary syndrome.

Triggering emotional activation seems to be more common

in people with low socio-economic status. The pathophysiological processes underlying trigger-ingcemotional has yet to be fully clarified but includes processes that can promote plaque rupture, together with a vascular prothrombotic environment which favors the formation of thrombi, and neuroendocrine and autonomic processes that stimulate rhythm disturbances.

For the moment, this knowledge has been used in clinical management to date, and the development of a systematic risk stratification and prevention must become a priority. Shortly it is also known about the frequency of triggers in the various ethnic groups, and it should also be stressed that women in many cohorts are underrepresented. However, the study of emotions as trigger promises important insights in favor of timing in managing acute cardiac events and opens up the possibility for new clinical management methods.

8.4 Clinical implications

Psychological interventions "evidence-based" have been developed for a long time in the field of cardiovascular rehabilitation, in order to empowerment coping resources, based on theoretical models derived from health psychology and psychotherapy cognitive behavior.

The cognitive-behavioral therapist, in fact, within a model

that postulates a complex relationship between emotions, thoughts, and behaviors, tries to help the patient to develop coping skills (the ability to cope with certain situations), through a series of techniques, including the development of the ability to speak to himself in a positive way (positive internal dialogue) and thus facilitate cognitive restructuring.

These techniques are already used worldwide by many of the psychologists working in cardiovascular rehabilitation; for example, stress management interventions, introduced for a long time in cardiovascular rehabilitation, were developed in the context of the interventions of cognitive-behavioral therapy.

The role of stress management in reducing the recurrence of major cardiovascular events is known and was recently confirmed by the results of a published study, which shows how cognitive-behavioral therapy is able to reduce events by 41% the fatal and non-fatal cardiovascular disease. In this randomized controlled trial, the researchers have assigned randomly 360 men and women who had been discharged from the hospital after an acute coronary event to the intervention group (conventional therapy and cognitive-behavioral therapy, n = 192) or to the usual care group, including the usual cardio-protection drug therapy (n = 170).

The program of cognitive-behavioral therapy, developed in

20 sessions of two hours each over the course of a year, is concentrated on reducing the experience of daily stress, on the urgency of time, and on the modification of hostility; it had five specific goals: education, self-monitoring, skills training, cognitive restructuring, and spiritual development.

The results, after an average follow-up of 94 months, have shown that the intervention group had a lower frequency of cardiovascular events, both fatal and non-fatal, fewer recurrences of acute myocardium heart attack, and an insignificant reduction in mortality from any cause.

Understanding the role of emotional stimuli as triggers in the onset of the acute coronary syndrome may instead lead to important clinical implications. Clinical strategies to reduce the risk of triggering should be integrated into the management of long-term risk factors. The vulnerability of emotional activation can expose some individuals to high risk when exposed people to interpersonal situations that arouse strong negative emotions.

If such individuals could be identified in advance, specific measures could be activated that include methods to reduce exposure to triggers, for example, anger management programs, addiction-awareness public campaigns, emergency programs, physical exercise programs, public outreach programs to highlight the potential danger of major sporting events, and strengthening social support to help people facing episodes of extreme sadness and depression stimulated by a mourning, losses and anniversaries, in addition to the already mentioned stress management programs.

In conclusion, it is certainly desirable that from care, prevention, and rehabilitation points of view, it is more and more expected that these patients are supported by a cardiologist and by a psychologist-psychotherapist that can identify subjects at higher risk and activating specific psychological interventions.

It is also fundamental for cardiologists to recognize the importance of psychosocial risk factors in relation to coronary heart disease, as they are often associated with this type of pathology. It is equally important that they put in place investigations, recognition, and management of these factors, because such strategies can lead to a reduced risk of developing atherosclerosis.

Furthermore, as previously mentioned, more attention should be paid to disclose prevention programs, especially among the population groups with the low socio-economic level of education.

Chapter 9 - Stress and eating disorders

9.1 Emotional Eating and Binge Eating

It can happen to eat not by hunger, but in response to feelings and emotions, particularly anger or stress. In these cases, we are faced with episodes of emotional eating, consisting of a loss of control, and the body no longer dictates what and how much to eat, but this is led by the emotions experienced at that moment.

Some people tend to binge when they are sad or particularly bored, for others it is a way to avoid thinking about delicate issues in their own lives. Emotional Eating often leads to overeating, especially foods with a high calorie and fat content, like sweets.

In cases where emotions affect the presence of repeated binges, we start facing a real disturbance, and we are talking about Binge Eating Disorder (BED) or Uncontrolled Eating Disorder, which is diagnosed in people who are usually overweight and who experience some specific symptoms, and this starts to be a common problem.

DSM-IV-TR diagnostic criteria for Uncontrolled Eating Disorder or BED (Binge Eating Disorder) are:

A. Recurrent episodes of uncontrolled feeding. An episode of uncontrolled feeding is characterized by the presence of both of the following elements:

   a. Eat, in a defined period of time (for example, within a period of 2 hours), a quantity of food clearly more abundant than most people would eat in a similar period of time and in similar circumstances;

   b. Feeling of loss of control in eating during the episode (for example, the feeling of not being able to stop or to control what and how much you are eating).

B. Uncontrolled feeding episodes are associated with three (or more) of the following symptoms:

   a. Eat faster than normal;

   b. Eat until you feel unpleasantly full;

   c. Eat large quantities of food even if you don't feel physically hungry;

   d. Eat alone because of the embarrassment of how much you are eating;

   e. Feeling disgusted, depressed, or very guilty after binge eating.

C. Present marked unease about uncontrolled eating.

    a. Uncontrolled feeding behavior occurs, on average, at least 2 days a week. Note: The method for determining the frequency is different from that used for nervous bulimia; future research should indicate whether the preferable method of identifying a threshold frequency either to count the number of days the binge eating occurs or to count the number of episodes of uncontrolled feeding over a 6-month period.

    b. Uncontrolled nutrition is not associated with the systematic use of inappropriate compensatory behavior (e.g., use of purgatives, fasting, excessive exercise), and it does not occur exclusively during nervous anorexia or nervous bulimia.

Regardless of whether all symptoms of the eating disorder are present, a considerable number of women admit episodes of BED. This subgroup of obese subjects presenting a BED shows more psychopathology, they often reach less results in weight-loss treatments, and they have a higher probability to go back to obesity if compared to non-BED subjects.

The BED is characterized by the consumption of high quantities of food and a sense of loose of control over eating. According to the Diagnostic and Statistical Manual of Mental Disorders (DSM-IV-TR), binge eating is defined, such as "eating large quantities of food in a reasonable period of time, accompanied by a sense of lack of control over eating." This is the characteristic symptom both of Nervous Bulimia (NB) and BED and can also be present in Nervous Anorexia (NA).

These individuals may also report a lack of control, vomiting, and other symptoms of clinical relevance (for example, food restrictions and concern for weight) even if they fail to meet the diagnostic criteria for NB and BED. Those individuals who do not meet the specific criteria for an eating disorder can experience significant discomfort with the behavior with food.

It is difficult to determine with certainty the prevalence of Binge Eating, because this behavior occurs as a symptom through a variety of clinical syndromes including NA, NB, obesity, and BED. In a 90s, research concluded that 25% of the female population admits behavior of Binge Eating, while 10% report at least one episode per week.

Using the QEWP questionnaire (Questionnaire on Eating and Weight Patterns) over 1650 subjects, it has been found that 9% of women and 5.2% of men reported Binge Eating at least once a week, and 26.6% of women declared themselves moderately to very distressed about the own eating behavior.

Emotional Eating is a way to eliminate or alleviate negative emotions, such as stress, anger, fear, boredom, sadness, and loneliness. Both important life events and controversies of everyday life can trigger negative emotions that bring the subject to let off steam on food; for example, unemployment, economic problems, health problems, conflicting relationships, stress at work, fatigue, etc., and food would only serve as a distraction.

Any emotion can lead to overeating, with the risk of entering a vicious cycle: whereby emotions lead to overeating and, subsequently, we feel downcast and guilty, and we eat again to deal with these negative emotions. Some of the most frequent emotions associated with Emotional Eating are:

1. Anger towards yourself, another person, or a situation; you tend to stifle feelings with food, rather than facing them;

2. Despair: it is thought that nothing will ever go well and therefore it is not worth to worry about health and weight;

3. Lack of control: you think you have no control over your life except for eating, so you think you can eat what you want and when you want;

4. Not feeling appreciated: no one notices the efforts made at work or in other areas of life;

5. Boredom: the person is bored, has nothing to do or places to go, he feels alone, and so he eats to fill those empty times.

Many theories have been proposed to explain Binge Eating, and some have included predisposing factors such as family functioning and peer relationships, sexual abuse, disturbed body image.

The most immediate antecedents were also considered, that is, events that predispose or increase motivation for behavior, such as cognitive events (e.g., an excess of concern for shape and weight), behavioral (e.g., diet or food restriction), and emotional (e.g., negative mood).

Some studies have shown that the prevalence of psychiatric diagnoses in subjects with Binge Eating Disorder is significantly higher than in the control group. It appears to be genetic components in the BED: the disorder has resulted associated with a melanocortin receptor mutation.

Additional supports for a biological basis of BED include physiological abnormalities in the actions of peripheral hormones such as insulin, leptin, and grieline. Other studies that looked at the relationship between eating disorders and behavioral coping skills have shown that women can acquire adaptive or maladaptive coping skills to deal with negative life events from family members, in particular by mothers and sisters (for example, modeling coping types through food or in the use of food as a positive reinforcement).

Some studies investigating the relationship between Binge Eating and coping made reference to the theory of escape from Binge Eating, whose premise is that binge eating reduces negative self-awareness. According to this theory, evasive coping strategies are widespread in groups of people with eating disorders.

Scholars suggest that in some studies, the avoidance-coping may have been confused with the level of depression. Also, the available measures of coping behavior do not evaluate effectively coping-evasive.

The factors that activate overeating have been called "disinhibitors" because they break down the self-imposed inhibition of eating. A classic disinhibitor is the presence of negative mood states. It has been well proven that negative emotions can be prior to an episode of Binge Eating. Anxiety, depression, boredom, anger, and loneliness have been cited as antecedents of binge eating in studies they investigated affective changes during binge eating and bulimic episodes.

It may seem that overeating or Binge Eating divert attention from the stressful event by focusing on other people or that overeat improves your mood in order to counteract the negative effects of stress on our mood itself.

Emotional triggers (feeling bored, depressed, anxious, sad, or tense) have all been reported as binge triggers in students who didn't have an eating disorder. It has been suggested that, in severely obese patients, alexithymic traits could reflect an underlying eating disorder (BED or Emotional Eating) as a result, a difficulty in reading internal stimuli.

Those studies confirmed that the induction of negative moods can push to overeat in dieters, but only when they declare the tendency to overindulge in food. On the contrary, women with a low restriction system, but high scores on the TFEQ disinhibition scale tend to eat more when they relax, and they tend to reduce their intake when under stress.

These results could partly explain past inconsistencies in the literature on nutrition induced by negative mood and/or stress and suggest that future studies cannot rely on the classification of participants on a solo basis of containment. This study also suggests that a positive mood can lead to overeating in women who are already prone in the absence of diet moderation, and it is desirable that future studies delve into the basics of such overeating in relation to obesity.

9.2 Stress and eating behavior

A growing number of studies show that stress affects health not only through direct physiological processes but also through changes in the behavior of health as a choice of foods and their intake. It seems obvious that stress is connected with nutrition. As we will see later, in fact, some research seems that stress alters the overall food intake in two ways, with an over- or under-feeding, depending on the severity of the stressful events.

Eating could also serve as a coping strategy (for example, as own escape) or be a means by which to reduce the adverse effects of high awareness of ourselves or even as a way to mitigate negative emotions induced by stress. Thus, it is possible for a certain eating behavior may serve both as an avoidance of emotions and as a possible coping strategy.

As noted by some scholars, the impact of stress can be both on the type of selected foods and on the amount of food consumed. It is a complex series of internal and external factors that influence the appetite and consequently, the quantity and type of food consumed by humans. Internal factors include physiological mechanisms that regulate appetite, with hormones such as the neuropeptide Y to stimulate intake of food and leptin to reduce food intake.

Among the external factors, we remember the environmental ones (for example, economic situation and food availability), social (for example, the influence of others) and the palatability of food products. Our body tries to keep its delicate and dynamic balance: any internal and external changes are compensated in order to maintain or restore homeostasis.

There is a growing amount of evidence from animal and human studies that suggests that a delay in prenatal growth can program a constantly hyperactive HPA axis in the fetus, which continues in childhood and even adulthood, and this can influence eating behaviors. In addition, this programming can be gender-specific, with an influencing prenatal growth adrenal cortical retardation responses to stress in boys and adrenal cortical activity baseline in girls.

Responses to acute or chronic stress can lead to physiological changes that include slowed gastric emptying, increased blood pressure and heart rate, mobilization of energy reserves, and reduction of blood flow to non-essential organs, for example, digestive system, kidneys, and skin.

Hormones released in response to stress can specifically affect appetite: norepinephrine and corticotropin have been reported to affect appetite suppression during stress, while cortisol is known to stimulate appetite during recovery from stress. Anxiety, depression, discomfort, anger, apathy, and alienation are emotions that commonly accompany chronic stress. Responses to acute or chronic stress also include a number of behavioral changes such as alcohol consumption, smoking, and eating.

9.3 The influence of stress on nutrition

One of the factors contributing to obesity can be the diet caused by stress, as it would result in a greater preference for nutritious foods, in particular those with high sugar and fat content. The effect of stress on the consumption of fats and sugars has been studied in humans.

In a large cross-sectional study involving more than 12000 people, it emerged that greater perceived stress was associated with a diet with a higher content of fats. In a study, individuals in situations with higher workload and perceived stress report increases in the total intake of energy and fat compared to periods with low workload and low perceived stress.

An American research has shown a prevalence of major obesity in African American subjects than in those of European origin, and obesity was found positively associated with the presence of stressors in African American women's lives. Further study has shown that African Americans seem to have a greater desire for sweet flavors and greater perception of stress compared to Americans of European origin.

This desire for sweet flavors could result in the choice and consumption of energy and nutrient foods and can be a contributing factor to the increased prevalence of obesity in that part of the population. The idea that stress can alter eating patterns is also widespread and, when acute stress is experienced as a threat to personal safety, there is an instantaneous physiological response to "flight or struggle," which translates into appetite suppression:

- Acute stress (e.g., threat to personal safety) -> Appetite decrease;

- Chronic psychological stress (e.g., work pressures) -> Consumption of highly energetic food.

Exposure to chronic psychological stressors, for example, as pressures at work, contributes to the overall disease burden and for many, the typical response to these chronic stress situations is not the avoidance of food but research and consumption of high energy density foods.

Obesity can be considered as a global epidemic, which is growing at an alarming rate, and it can be attributed to a myriad of genetic and environmental factors.

If stress causes some individuals to consume excess food, then this can lead to weight gain and obesity. There are models according to which there are two ways in which stress can affect nutrition, with consequences of over- or under-nutrition. These contrary responses can be explained by the severity of the stresses encountered.

Human studies have shown in some cases a decrease and in other cases an increase in nutrition habits in response to stress depending on the severity of the stressful factor, as well as personal characteristics of the subjects. A study on food intake by the U.S. Marines during a fight provided an opportunity to examine the effect of a highly stressful situation on eating behavior.

During the first day of combat, 68% Marines said they eat less than usual. The main reason given is the lack of time, followed by fear, which included "being nervous, tense and frightened." In a prospective study, 160 male and female subjects completed 86 daily reports on stress: subjects reported both decrease and increase in nutrition in response to stress. Moreover, the probability of eating less increased with the greater severity of the stress factors.

The effects of self-reported stress on eating behavior have been tested on 200 students, and it was found that about an equal number of subjects reported eating more (42%) and to eat less (38%), but it was not reported any information on the influence of the severity of the stressors.

In another study, it has been investigated the effect of a major stressful event (for example, a school exam) on food consumption in 230 high school students.

The total energy intake was significantly higher on the day of the exam if compared with a stress-free day (2300 Kcal versus 2080 kcal, respectively). In another work, the effect of a mild stress factor (movie) was assessed on food consumption: in general, the group of males subjected to stress consumed a significantly lower amount of food than the male control group (respectively 100 against 238 kcal). Furthermore, no difference in food consumption was detected between female gender groups, which indicates that gender can influence behavior on food intake after mild stress. Stress can also increase or decrease food intake in humans, although it is difficult to determine whether the severity of the stress has a role, because few studies are available, which are characterized by a series of limits, including the use of inaccurate methods for measuring food intake.

An alternative explanation of why calorie intake is higher during stressful life periods may not be linked to the stress itself, but rather to the insufficient time to buy and prepare food and the increased use of ready-made foods, which are generally highly energetic. There are few studies that have measured the effect of stress induced in the laboratory, on the selection of food.

Subjects of both sexes subjected to an acute stress factor (like preparing a speech) have consumed similar quantities of sweet foods compared to a control group. In another study, premenopausal women did not change their food intake habits, including desserts with fat content, even if subjected to 45 minutes of stress (visual-spatial puzzles, serial subtraction of a prime number from a large number, and the delivery of a videotaped intervention), compared with subjects in non-stress condition.

The researchers found that subjects with increased levels of salivary cortisol significantly consumed a higher number of calories (225 versus 145 kcal) and a greater quantity of sweet and high fat content foods on stressed days compared to low stressed ones.

The data collected in various research suggests that the foods selected by individuals who respond to stress by eating more are typically high in sugar and fats. Although there are few published studies in this area, there is evidence that chronic life stress is associated with a higher fat diet and a higher preference for sweet foods.

Some scholars have pointed out the limits of the studies examined, including the use of a suboptimal method for measuring levels of stress and too few samples. In addition, artificial stress created in an environment may not be high enough to change food behavior, thus making the evaluation of the effects on a preference for certain nutrients unreliable in laboratory studies.

In a large cross-sectional study on workers in Finland (37,000 women and 9,000 men) there was a weak association between work stress and body mass index (BMI,). It emerged that stress-related nutrition (defined in research as trying, in a stressful situation to feel better by eating or drinking) was significantly associated with obesity only in women and not in men.

This can be a gender specific response to stress: women are more likely to use food to deal with stress, while men are more likely to use other behaviors like alcohol consumption or smoking as strategies to face stress.

If stress-induced nutrition contributes to the development of obesity, then obese individuals would be expected to consume more food in response to stress compared to thin subjects. Two studies measured the effect of stress in daily life, and three others induced stress in an artificial setting. Among these five studies, two reported an increase in the consumption of food in obese subjects.

It would also be reasonable to expect obese individuals to consume more food to maintain weight; however, in one of these studies in which the usual food consumption and perceived stress were recorded (pleasant, neutral, or unpleasant) in women of normal weight and overweight for over 4 months, it emerged that in overweight women the total food intake was not found associated with the daily stress level, while normal weight women have eaten more on pleasant days. Therefore, there is no clear evidence that food intake increases with chronic stress in obese people.

The effect of stressful life events on BMI change over a period of 6 months has been studied in subjects classified as High Emotional Eater (i.e., who respond to stress by eating more) or Low Emotional Eater (which respond to stress by eating less). It turned out that only the male subjects have responded to stress by increasing food consumption reported more than three life stressful events and have had weight gain during the 6 months.

High starting levels of stress have seen a 10 kg weight gain over a period of 6 years in men but not in women, showing that an increase in work stress has also increased the risk of weight in 5 years in those subjects with a higher body mass index, and loss of weight in thin people, and this bidirectional effect observed between work stress and BMI was observed only in men and not in women.

All these studies together suggest that higher stress levels likely increase to gain weight, with a greater effect in men than in women. It can be concluded that stress is positively correlated with body weight, even if these results should be interpreted with caution, because they are based on measures of weight and height self-reported by the subjects, which can be the cause of bias.

Only a few studies have been able to properly measure the effects on humans of stress induced in the laboratory or in real-life contexts and have demonstrated the presence of a significant increase in food consumption in obese subjects. It is not possible to detect effects from acute stress induced in the laboratory because individuals may not be sufficiently stressed in this artificial environment compared to the stress experienced in the real world.

Furthermore, it must be remembered that laboratory studies can only measure the effect of acute stress and not chronic stress, which could have a greater effect on behavior with food. The laboratory environment allows strict control of food intake. Longitudinal studies are the most useful for investigating the effect of chronic life stress on eating behavior, but precise nutrition data can be difficult to harvest for long periods.

There also seems to be an association between chronic life stress and weight gain in the future, with a greater effect in men than in women, although the reason for this difference is unclear. In examining this relationship, it is important to consider the two sides of the energy balance equation: intake and expenditure.

In all the studies cited, these two factors were not measured, therefore, it is not known whether the reported weight gain is caused by an increase in intake energy or from a decrease in physical activity levels. Regarding the relationship between stress and physical activity levels, while two studies do not have reported any association, one has shown that physical activity levels decrease in a period of stress.

Despite the limitations highlighted, some general conclusions can be drawn in support of the idea that stress can affect food intake. The studies examined revealed that stress can lead to both a decrease and an increase in nutrition. These behaviors may be related to the severity of stressors: severe stress in mice results in a lower intake, while in humans, the response is variable. Studies suggest that high levels of stress are associated with an increased desire for highly palatable foods rich in energy. This can contribute to excessive energy intake and weight gain.

9.3.1 The role of cortisol

Cortisol is involved in regulating appetite and energy balance, increasing the energy available through gluconeogenesis and lipolysis. The relationship between cortisol and eating behavior has been studied more frequently in mice than in men. However, studies have shown that in healthy males, the administration of exogenous glucocorticoids increases the daily intake of food compared to the placebo group.

A further indication of cortisol's involvement in weight

regulation is the similarity observed between hypercortisolism and obesity. Patients with Cushing's syndrome, characterized by high levels of cortisol, choose foods with a high content of fat in double measure in comparison to the subjects of normal weight, and three times more often overweight control subjects. In Cushing's syndrome, it is common to have weight gain with abdominal fat distribution, among other symptoms of obesity.

In the Night Eating Syndrome, the nocturnal elevation of cortisol could help induce awakenings to eat. Only one study looked at both the changes in cortisol and food intake following a laboratory stressor, and it found that among healthy women, those with a greater reaction to cortisol, they ate significantly more food after a stressful cognitive task compared to those with low cortisol reaction.

In summary, after a stressful cognitive task:

- Healthy women with high reaction to cortisol -> Increase of food behavior;

- Healthy women with low reaction to cortisol -> No variations in food behavior.

To date, no studies have examined cortisol and food intake in obese subjects with BED. Direct observations of cortisol involvement in weight gain are recently presented in a case-control study. This study has compared women who gained weight after a stressful event with women in whom the development of obesity was not due to stress and women in the control group with a weight in the norm.

There were no differences in urine free cortisol between the control group with normal weight and the group with obesity unconnected to stress, but cortisol had increased significantly in the group of subjects with stress-related obesity.

Exaggerated cortisol responses to stress have been observed in women with nervous anorexia (NA), nervous bulimia (NB), and obesity. Few studies have looked at the long-term stress response to cortisol, although higher values have been observed of 24-hour urinary cortisol in women with BN the day after a task (which consisted of interpersonal discourse) compared to a control group.

Only one study has failed to observe the rise in cortisol levels as a result of a stressful mental challenge test in the NB, despite the higher basic levels compared to a control group of healthy subjects. In this study - the first to examine cortisol following BED stress - was found a tendency to increase the circulating cortisol in BED subjects compared to non-BED subjects, as a consequence of Cold Pressor Test not linked to depression score.

The weight gain of the group with obesity linked to stress is greater and in a significantly shorter period of time. These results suggest that an increase in cortisol levels is involved in the development of obesity rather than the other way round.

Several studies have analyzed the role of stress and cortisol in food intake. In a survey carried out through a questionnaire submitted to male Japanese workers, obesity was associated with dysfunctional eating behavior and linked to high demands for work, tiredness, depression, and anxiety.

In a recent study, it has been given to healthy people, the hormone that releases corticotropin (CRH), which has caused the increase of the secretion of cortisol, which resulted in an increase in food consumption and intake of calories in the participants.

These results support the observation that stress increases the intake of snacks in people with high cortisol levels and, therefore, these results connect the stress system to the regulation of food intake.

It can be summarized that the cortisol can act on food intake and on the choice of food through different mechanisms:

- inducing leptin resistance and, therefore, blocking the suppressive effects of intake leptin food, and/or

- Increasing the release of the neuropeptide Y (NPY) which stimulates the adipose production of tissue. NPY release was characterized in a model with animals in which the induced stress increased both the release of NPY and the growth of abdominal fat. Interestingly, this effect of NPY appears to be at least partially as a function of glucocorticoids (i.e., cortisol in human beings).

Since stress usually leads to an increase in energy expenditure, these cortisol mechanisms (leptin and NPY) can contribute physiologically in keeping the total energy content of the body relatively constant.

There is no reliable evidence that cortisol can influence appetite regulation through NPY and leptin, however, cortisol increases appear to be followed by a high secretion of NPY and dulling of the leptin system (food inhibitory arm); so the overall effect can be an increase in intake of food.

The above studies seem to all point in the same direction: with different approaches and methodologies, show that the stress system and cortisol release can be a cause of obesity, thus representing mechanisms started before the increase of weight. This is supported by the idea that visceral obesity can be considered as a physiological adaptation to stress.

It appears that although an acute elevation of cortisol plays a protective role during stress, persistently high levels promote insulin resistance and abdominal obesity. Stress reactions have been associated with the development of abdominal obesity. It has been proposed that the repeated activation of the hypothalamic-pituitary adrenal (HPA) axis for stress, with the consequent increase in cortisol, leads to the activation of lipase of the lipoprotein of the adipose tissue and, therefore, to the accumulation of abdominal fat mass.

Secretion of stress-induced cortisol was mostly observed in men and women with abdominal obesity, but it is not clear whether obesity is responsible for the highest levels of cortisol in case of stress or if the highest cortisol level leads to obesity.

Many studies have observed that chronic stress overactive the HPA axis and feeds the release of insulin, which in turn activates the storage of abdominal fat. However, the literature is mixed, in the sense that some studies show a slow response of the HPA axis to awakening in men with higher abdominal fat.

The distribution of abdominal fat also appears to be linked to vulnerability to stress. For example, in response to laboratory stress, women with a high waist-hip ratio report feeling more threatened and have higher reactivity to cortisol compared to women with a low waist-hip ratio.

Another study on overweight women found a positive correlation between cortisol levels following the Cold Pressor Test (CPT) and the sagittal diameter of the belly. It has been observed a relationship between waist-hip ratio and levels of cortisol following CPT only in women with BED. This relationship persisted even after 6 weeks of treatment consisting of a liquid diet and a cognitive-behavioral path.

It can be concluded that stress is positively correlated with body weight, although these results must be interpreted with caution, because they are based on measures of weight and height self-reported by the subjects, which can be the cause of bias.

We repeat that only a few studies focused on humans subjected to stress in the laboratory or in real-life contexts have been able to measure the effect of stressful life events and have demonstrated the presence of a significant increase in food consumption in obese subjects. It is not possible to detect effects from inducing acute stress in the laboratory because individuals may not be sufficiently stressed in this artificial environment compared to the stress experienced in the real world.

Furthermore, it must be remembered that laboratory studies can only measure the effect of acute stress and not chronic stress, which could have a greater effect on food behavior. The laboratory environment allows strict control on food intake, while longitudinal studies are the most effective for investigating the effect of chronic stress on eating behavior, but precise nutrition data can be difficult to harvest for long periods.

Responses to acute stress are associated with physiological changes that could be expected to reduce short-term food intake, for example, slowed gastric emptying and transit of blood from the gastrointestinal tract to the muscles. In other situations, however, chronic stress causes a more passive response driven by the HPA axis, with increases in cortisol, which can lead people to consume energy-dense foods and potentially can produce an unwanted weight gain and obesity.

We must also remember that cortisol can contribute to the accumulation of abdominal fat mass. Most of the studies quantify stress using only subjective measurements. Some physiological measurements of stress could be included in future studies to measure cortisol and catecholamine levels. Studies on animals could identify some links between stress hormones and neurotransmitters regulating appetite, which should help us understand the mechanisms and to undertake preventive treatments.

9.3.2 Does obesity affect the level of stress?

Obesity can be considered as a potential stress inducer on

the body. In an experiment of the early 70s, in some men who deliberately have increased their body fat mass, some increased cortisol levels were measured. These observations have most recently been confirmed by a study on elderly and middle-aged men, which showed how the cortisol increase appears to be dependent on weight gain. These two studies show that the increase in cortisol can be secondary to weight gain and not a cause:

Increase of weight -> Stress -> Cortisol increase

However, it may not be as evident that obesity activates the response to stress. Two independent studies suggest that cortisol release increases secondary to weight gain. However, we must remember that studies that report an increase in cortisol following weight gain are limited. One of the two studies is based on intentional augmentation experiments of body mass, which may not exactly represent the spontaneous development of obesity.

The other study must be accepted with caution due to the finding that age-related weight loss and not weight gain has been associated with increased cortisol levels.

One of the characteristics of obesity is chronic low-grade inflammation in which adipose tissues release various inflammatory mediators, including interleukin (IL)-1, IL-6, and the tumor necrosis factor alpha (TNF-alpha). These three pro-inflammatory cytokines are able to activate the

HPA axis autonomously or together, thus increasing the release of cortisol in an attempt to limit the inflammatory reaction. So there is a pathophysiological link between obesity, activation of inflammation, and release of cortisol that could be relevant in the regulation of stress response in obese people.

Another feature of obesity is the increase in secretion, and the high levels of leptin, a hormone that could play a key role in the development and also in obesity therapy. Leptin secretion and the HPA axis appear to be functionally connected under physiological conditions. In experiments on healthy individuals, cortisol has been shown to increase leptin levels, and this increase of leptin has increased cortisol levels. Thus, the increase in leptin levels, as it occurs in obesity, can trigger the increase of cortisol release.

9.3.3 The role of depression

In mammals, the primary stress response systems are glucocorticoids and catecholamine, and the release of these molecules from the adrenal glands into the blood in response to stressful stimuli is manifested in rapid and postponed alterations in cardiovascular, immune, and metabolic functions. These changes, in turn, promote survival by directing the flow of energy to the directly responsible systems to deal with the threat, while promoting the suppression of other systems competing for energy resources.

The endocannabinoid system, which exists both in the brain and in the periphery, is not only a regulator but also an effector of the stress response. This system is involved in multiple control and adaptation systems of the organism. In general, it has a rebalancing function in the body as a response to disturbances or stress. For example, during a prolonged fast, due, for example, to skipping a meal, the system activates and produces hunger stimuli to stimulate intake of food and bring the body back into balance. At that point, the endocannabinoid system deactivates. Unfortunately, an incorrect diet rich in fat causes an increase in the activity of the endocannabinoid system in the hypothalamus.

As a consequence of this, constantly high levels of endocannabinoids cause a greater desire to eat energetic foods by creating gratification from the food itself but also a dangerous vicious circle, where the system continues to be activated, which in turn perpetuates excessive nutrition:

> High-fat diet -> increased activity of the endocannabinoid system -> Elevated levels of endocannabinoids -> Greater desire to eat energy foods -> High-fat diet-> etc., etc.

This vicious circle leads to obesity and related disorders

such as diabetes, increased fat in the blood, hypertension, and atherosclerosis. The prolonged increase in endocannabinoids also increases the ability to store fat aside by adipose cells, contributing to obesity. Preclinical studies have shown that the content of endocannabinoids in limbic and rhomboencephalon regions are regulated by a variety of stressful stimuli.

These changes in endocannabinoid activity dampen or promote the recovery of the hormonal response to stress after the endocannabinoid response inhibited the hypothalamic-pituitary-adrenal (HPA) axis. From a functional point of view, peripheral endocannabinoids are known to modulate metabolic processes (adipose-genesis, blood glucose levels), cardiovascular processes (vasoconstriction and blood pressure), and immune processes (production of pro- and anti-inflammatory).

All these physiological processes are influenced in a coordinated way by exposure to stress. Studies have shown that the endocannabinoid content in the blood is significantly reduced in subjects with major depression and that physiological responses related to inflammatory processes and metabolic disorders are impaired in subjects suffering from depressive illness. Data show that the exposure of humans to an acute social stress factor impairs circulating endocannabinoid concentrations.

In depressed women, it has experienced a reduction in the

production of a particular endocannabinoid, anandamide (AEA). It has been hypothesized that perhaps the AEA synthesis pathway is interrupted in depressed women, leading to a reduction in this endocannabinoid, but not in others (e.g., PEA or OEA). However, the mechanism by which these levels decrease in the major depression currently remains uncertain.

Given the physiological role of endocannabinoids, it seems reasonable to assume that this reduction of circulating levels of endocannabinoids in depression may be associated with increased inflammation, cardiovascular disease, and auto-immune dysfunction that can be found in this disease. Endocannabinoids are also known to affect mood and emotions, so much that impairments in endocannabinoid signaling can produce depression and anxiety.

Consequently, the endocannabinoid deficiency in circulation in documented subjects with major depression can contribute to the emotional sequelae associated with this same disease. Preclinical studies indicate that the central content of endocannabinoids is regulated by glucose-corticoid hormones that are released in response to stress.

Women were exposed to stress in the morning, when cortisol is at its diurnal peak, and this prevents the detection of an increase of salivary cortisol as a consequence of exposure to stress. Thus, the increase of endocannabinoid cannot be explained by an increase in glucose-corticoids.

In the future, it would be interesting to examine whether changes in endocannabinoid values induced by stress may be involved in other physiological changes evoked by exposure to stress. Considered the role of endocannabinoids in the regulation of appetite and metabolism it is of particular interest to determine if there is a role of endocannabinoids in the stress-induced food intake, in the accumulation of fat and, potentially, in obesity and metabolic syndrome.

9.3.4 Positive reciprocal interactions between stress and obesity?

Together, the studies presented here show that:

- Stress as a cause of obesity seems a well-established theory; and

- Stress as a consequence of obesity is less documented, but is still probable and maybe dependent on gender.

It seems evident that stress can cause obesity. This is demonstrated by several observations, including:

- Similarities between hypercortisolism and the characteristics of obesity;

- Differences between stress-induced and non-stress induced weight gain;

- Weight gain in depressed people;

- Changes in food consumption due to stress and cortisol.

These observations suggest that stress induces weight gain, such as examined in depth in various studies. In addition, a greater activity of 11Beta-HSD1, the activation of inflammations, as well as the increase in leptin secretion, they can indirectly affect the activation of the stress system in obese people. Several mechanisms thus have the potential to influence the stress system in obese people.

Interestingly, the energy restriction in obese people increases cortisol secretion, highlighting the complexity between obesity and response to stress, but also showing that the increase in the release of cortisol and stress can be secondary to obesity, for example, during strict diets. Cortisol levels are not increased in women with a non-induced obesity from stress.

However, this figure can be explained by different

mechanisms. An explanation may be the normal biological variability: the simple fact that different people have different reaction patterns. The latter point, combined with the relatively low number of participants (stress-induced obesity, n = 15; non-stress-induced obesity, n = 22), may have influenced the study outcome. Another possible and interesting explanation is that due to gender differences.

In this study on stress-induced or non-stressed obesity, only women were observed, while studies that showed an increase in secondary cortisol in line with weight gain included only men. The differences of gender have also been observed in a study of depressed adolescents, in which the link between depression and body mass index (BMI) mediated by the reactivity of cortisol was significant only for girls.

Gender differences in the HPA axis activities in obesity are well known and seem to involve a gender hormone imbalance, so differences in obesity seem likely to depend on gender.

Therefore, it seems possible that stress is potentially a cause and consequence of obesity, interacting in a bidirectional model. This means that weight gain has the potential to trigger the stress response that, in turn, can increase weight, and so on in a dangerous vicious circle.

Likewise, weight loss, which can also trigger the release of cortisol, could trigger the response to stress and, therefore, further oppose weight loss, which suggests that the stress system can be involved in weight loss challenges.

This model with positive feedback between stress and obesity indicates that the treatment of obesity should not only focus on the energy balance, but also on the stress system and its stressors. In order to break the spiral between stress and obesity, it may be important to identify and remove possible stressors.

This would not only be a positive factor for weight reduction but also to improve the quality of life. Further studies of the interaction between obesity and stress are necessary to fully understand the causes of obesity.

9.3.5 Limitations of studies conducted to date

There are several limitations in the studies conducted to date on stress and food behavior food. Researchers use a variety of methods to induce stress in the laboratory, and therefore it is difficult to compare the results between the various studies. None of the approaches used are naturalistic, and therefore these studies do not reveal anything about the factors that can actually lead to Binge Eating in real life.

Furthermore, these laboratory stressors have different

durations, from 2 to 45 minutes. The psychological factors of eating disorders in humans have been more widely studied with respect to biological factors. Most of the studies have measured food intake resulting from laboratory stressors without measuring the biological correlates.

Surprisingly, many cases have observed no differences in general levels of consumption, but rather differences in the content of macronutrients. For example, it has been found no difference between women with bulimic symptoms and women in the control group following a task of interpersonal speech. However, both bulimic women and those of the control group increased carbohydrate consumption after stressful activity compared to the stress-free control condition.

Furthermore, it has been observed an increase in ice cream consumption following the stressful task and after viewing of scary movies compared to a day of inspection, but consumption did not differ between normal weight subjects affected by Binge Eating and those not characterized by normal behavior.

Only in one case, a laboratory study examined stress and intake of food in BED subjects and found no difference in calories ingested during a buffet compared to the control group following the induction of a negative mood compared to neutral mood. Emotional eating has been associated with both an increase and a decrease in food intake, and little is known about the mechanisms underlying the management of change.

Typically, stress responses cause anorexia and, if the effort is persistent enough, weight loss. The long-term vision is that stress produces sympathetic excitement, which results in a reduction rather than an increase in nutrition. It is unclear why some men show opposite reactions in eating behavior when faced with stress. As previously mentioned, the direction of change in consumption can be expected from withheld eating habits. People on a diet turned out more likely to report stress hyperphagia, and they are more likely to report stress hypophagy.

There is strong evidence that both sober eaters and emotional eaters eat too much in response to stress. Emotional eaters respond to stressors eating more sweets, high-fat foods, and more meals with high energy density compared to non-stressed and non-emotional eaters.

Eating behavior is complex and multifaceted, and the reactivity to stress, both physiological and psychological, can distinguish the subjects who eat more by those who eat less. A more sophisticated understanding of these mechanisms has not been extensively studied, and further experiments should be put in place to better understand the relationship between stress and nutrition.

The integration of these factors is fundamental to understand obesity and Binge Eating from a biopsychosocial perspective, which could contribute to better treatment options for those patients who experience marked psychological distress and impairment.

9.3.6 Evaluation tools for BED and Emotional Eating

The development of psychometric assessments of eating behavior has focused around three main theories:

1. Psychosomatic theory, focused on overeating, in response to negative emotional cues;

2. Theory of externality, which describes the tendency to eat in response to hedonic stimuli regardless of the internal state of hunger or satiety.

3. Theory of withholding, in which external and emotional eating, is postulated to be a consequence of a diet.

In this research, the currently developed tools have focused on the two main food behavior theories that have proven to be more consistently associated with body weight: psychosomatic theory and the theory of externality.

Some of these tools used in the researches to measurement

of BED and Emotional Eating are briefly illustrated:

- Tool: EDI-2; Scale: Bulimia; Items: 7;

- Tool: Restraint scale; Scale: Weight fluctuation, Diet Concern; Items: 10;

- Tool: TFEQ; Scale: Cognitive control; Disinhibition, Hunger; Items: 51;

- Tool: RC-FC scale; Scale: Rigid control, Flexible control; Items: 28;

- Tool: DEBQ; Scale: Restriction, Emotional eating, Overfeeding for external stimuli; Items: 33;

- Tool: WREQ; Scale: Compensatory withholding, Routine withholding, Susceptibility to external stimuli, Emotional Eating; Items: 16.

Inventory-2 (EDI-2) can be used to evaluate the behaviors of Binge Eating. This subscale is made up of 7 items and focuses mainly on the desire to think and/or engage in Binge Eating behaviors. The psychometric property of the Bulimia scale of EDI-2 are excellent.

Moreover, EDI-2 has shown good convergent and discriminating validity among female university students. High correlations have also been found between this subscale and the "Bulimia and Food Concern" scale of EAT-26.

In the 70s, the Restraint Scale (RS), the first dietary restriction measure, was developed and subsequently revised in the 80s; while RS has been a widely used measure, construction and predictive validity of this tool have been criticized for references to fluctuation weight and concentration on the diet, and its inability to predict patterns food, especially of obese individuals.

To improve the validity of the RS, in the mid-eighties, two other tools on eating behaviors have been developed: the Three Factor Eating Questionnaire (TFEQ), consisting of 51 items, and the Dutch Eating Van Strien's Behavior Questionnaire (DEBQ) consisting of 33 items. The TFEQ is a self-report tool that contains three different subscales:

- Cognitive containment, the measure of efforts made to limit food intake;

- Disinhibition, the exploration of the tendency to lose control over the consumption of food;

- Hunger, the recording of subjects' susceptibility to feel hunger in relationship to environmental food stimuli.

The DEBQ measures external and emotional nutrition. In an attempt to perfect the measure of the dietetics restriction, it has been observed that the restriction scales of TFEQ (TFEQ-R) and DEBQ (DEBQ-R) evaluate a different aspect of the restriction system: while it has been demonstrated that RS predicts uninhibited nutrition and has a positive association with Binge Eating, TFEQ-R and DEBQ-R were predictive of reduced energy intake and have negative associations with Binge Eating.

Exploring the conceptual differences between limitations measured by RS and TFEQ-R, two subscales of restriction have been introduced on the basis of inverse associations with disinhibition: rigid control (RC) and flexible control (FC). RC is characterized as a dichotomy – approach "all or nothing" to food, "weight control or binge eating" - and it shows positive correlations with the BMI.

FC represents instead an approach with minor profile, routine, to control weight and has negative associations with BMI. To evaluate RC and CF and improve interpretative functionality of the original TFEQ-R, an RC-FC scale of 28 items was developed and validated. Currently, however, there is no measure that collectively evaluates the multiple aspects of restriction in eating behavior associated with disinhibition.

Since TFEQ and DEBQ have been designed to integrate psychosomatic theory and externality theory, the questionnaires have items that reflect the concept of active overconsumption. However, there is no element in both questionnaires, which clearly reflects passive overconsumption.

The new Weight-Related Eating Questionnaire (WREQ) measures four constructs:

- Withholding holding (WREQ-CR) and ordinary holding (WREQ-RR), which represent the Dietary Restraint theory;

- Susceptibility to external stimuli (WREQ-EX), which represents the theory of externality;

- Emotional Eating (WREQ-EE) which represents the psychosomatic theory.

WREQ-CR is defined as the intentional limitation of energy intake after an overeating episode. WREQ-RR is defined as the routine perception of restriction of energy intake to control weight. WREQ-EX postpones eating in response to sensorial signals, without regard for internal signals of hunger or satiety. WREQ-EE refers to eating in response to negative emotions. The WREQ shows a strong convergent validity with the corresponding scales of similar tools on eating behavior. Although there is strong similarity to existing tools, the WREQ is unique as it allows individual evaluations of two food restraint subscales (WREQ-RR and WREQ-CR).